PEPTIDE POWER

Clinically proven strategies to burn fat, build lean muscle, relieve joint pain, rejuvenate skin, and extend healthy lifespan

JULIAN CROSS

Disclaimer

- Introduction

This publication is intended for informational and educational purposes only. The author and publisher are not providing medical, legal, fitness, or other professional advice. Nothing in this work should be relied upon as a substitute for qualified professional consultation. Always seek the guidance of a licensed healthcare provider, attorney, or other qualified professional before acting on any information contained herein.

- No Advice

The content in this book does not constitute medical, legal, or professional advice. You should never act, or refrain from acting, based solely on the material presented here without obtaining professional guidance specific to your individual circumstances.

- Assumption of Risk

By reading and applying the material in this book, you acknowledge that participation in any practices, strategies, or protocols described involves inherent risks. You voluntarily assume full responsibility for any outcomes, including physical, financial, or other consequences, that may result from the use or misuse of the information provided.

- Indemnification

You agree to indemnify, defend, and hold harmless the author, publisher, affiliates, and their respective officers, employees, agents, and licensors from and against any claims, liabilities, damages, losses, costs, or expenses (including reasonable attorneys' fees) that may arise from your use of this book, your violation of these terms, or your infringement of the rights of others.

- No Representations or Warranties

The author and publisher make no representations or warranties of any kind, express or implied, regarding the completeness, accuracy, reliability, or suitability of the information provided. All content is offered "as is", without any warranty of merchantability, fitness for a particular purpose, or non-infringement.

- Limitation and Exclusion of Liability

To the fullest extent permitted by law, the author, publisher, and affiliates shall not be liable for any direct, indirect, incidental, consequential, or special damages, including but not limited to personal injury, loss of profits, loss of data, or business interruption, arising from your use of this book or inability to use its contents, even if advised of the possibility of such damages.

- Severability

If any provision of this disclaimer is found invalid, unlawful, or unenforceable by a court of competent jurisdiction, that provision shall be severed, and the remaining provisions shall remain valid and enforceable to the fullest extent permitted by law.

- Governing Law and Jurisdiction

This disclaimer and any disputes arising from it shall be governed by and construed in accordance with the laws of the State of Missouri, without regard to conflict of law principles. You agree to submit to the exclusive jurisdiction of the state and federal courts located in St. Louis County, Missouri for the resolution of any disputes.

Table of Contents

Introduction — 5

Chapter 1: Peptides Unlocked: What They Are and Why They Work — 6

Chapter 2: The Language of Life: How Peptides Talk to Your Cells — 20

Chapter 3: The Fat-Loss Reset: Why Diets Fail and How Peptides Restart Metabolism — 37

Chapter 4: Lean Muscle Power: Rebuild Strength, Protect Metabolism, and Age Strong — 58

Chapter 5: Joint & Pain Repair Power: Heal, Move Better, and Stay Active for Life — 71

Chapter 6: Skin, Hair & Beauty from the Inside Out: Collagen Renewal for Visible Vitality — 82

Chapter 7: Sleep, Energy & Mood Reset Power: Reclaim Calm, Focus & Deep Recovery — 105

Chapter 8: Gut, Immunity & Inflammation Control: The Core of Longevity — 116

Chapter 9: Stack Mastery Guide: Build Your Custom Plan with Confidence — 123

Chapter 10: The Power Lifestyle System: Make Results Automatic — 129

Chapter 11: Safety, Sourcing & Stacking the Smart Way — 140

Chapter 12: The 30-Day Power Reset Blueprint — 149

Chapter 13: Sustain & Expand: How to Keep Results for Life — 156

Bonus: Unlock Your Power Toolkit — 165

Conclusion: Awaken Your Power Wellness — 166

References — 170

INTRODUCTION

When you've done everything right, clean eating, consistent workouts, supplements, and progress still stalls, it's not your discipline that's broken. It's your internal communication. Deep within your body is a network that coordinates how you burn fat, build muscle, recover, and stay mentally sharp. When those biological signals weaken, your results plateau, your energy dips, and your motivation fades. The key isn't to push harder, it's to help your body remember how to talk to itself again. That's where peptides come in.

Peptides are like the body's native language, tiny messengers that restore clear communication between your cells. Instead of forcing change, they guide your system back to its optimal rhythm.

Here's what reactivating your internal signal system can do for you:

- Trigger natural fat burning instead of forced restriction
- Support muscle repair and recovery for lasting strength
- Rebuild collagen and joint tissue for smoother movement
- Reduce inflammation and accelerate recovery cycles
- Enhance focus, mood, and cognitive clarity
- Promote long-term vitality through balance and precision

Peptide Power is not about hype or shortcuts. It's a strategy built on awareness, alignment, and sustainable chemistry. Once your body starts communicating clearly again, progress stops feeling like a battle, and starts feeling like balance restored.

Welcome to **Peptide Power**, where science becomes strategy, and your best results finally make sense.

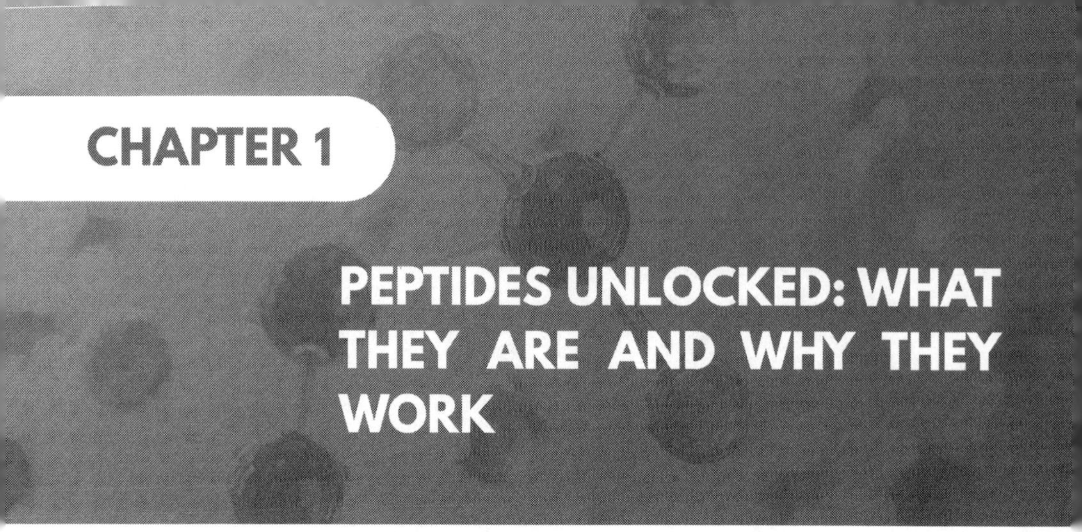

CHAPTER 1

PEPTIDES UNLOCKED: WHAT THEY ARE AND WHY THEY WORK

The New Science of Renewal

Modern life, characterized by endless work, poor sleep, processed foods, and constant stress, has severely tested our physical and mental health. We constantly chase new diets and supplements that promise to fix what feels broken. The missing piece is not trying harder, but restoring how the body communicates internally. The body operates as a network of messages, and when communication weakens, energy, recovery, focus, mood decline, and aging accelerates. Peptides reconnect this broken network by working in harmony with your biology, helping your body remember how to repair, renew, and function optimally.

Key Insights

- **Modern health under pressure:** Fast-paced lifestyles and poor habits have weakened the body's ability to recover and perform.
- **Why typical fixes don't last:** Quick solutions like strict diets or potent supplements often push the body too hard without addressing the deeper issue of communication.
- **The real missing link, "communication":** Clear **cellular communication** is essential for every biological process. Weakened signals negatively affect energy, metabolism, and aging.
- **What peptides do:** Peptides act as messengers, sending specific instructions to cells to help coordinate natural repair, growth, and regeneration.

- **How peptides differ from stimulants or drugs:** Instead of forcing a reaction, peptides gently "whisper instructions" for healing, restoring balance, and optimizing function.
- **The precision advantage:** Peptide therapy is highly **targeted**, focusing on specific processes like fat loss, muscle recovery, inflammation control, and energy renewal.
- **From elite science to everyday wellness:** Peptides, once limited to clinical research, are now gaining popularity in mainstream wellness due to their safe and natural effectiveness. They represent a quiet revolution that awakens the body by restoring natural communication. The goal is to unlock the body's existing potential, not adding more to the routine.

Why This Chapter Matters

Finding true health shouldn't feel complicated. If you are **past 35**, you have likely tried numerous diets and plans that left you confused. What is truly needed is **understanding**. Knowing *why* something works makes consistent, lasting progress easier. This chapter is designed to give you that "aha" moment, serving as a guide to understanding how peptides naturally **optimize performance** without pushing the body beyond its limits.

What You'll Learn in This Chapter

- **Clear understanding of peptides:** Discover what peptides are and how they function in the body's communication system.
- **The safety factor:** Learn why peptides are considered safer and more targeted than many traditional supplements or hormone therapies.
- **Precision in action:** See how peptides support specific functions, such as fat burning, muscle building, and recovery, through natural cellular signaling.
- **Whole-body benefits:** Understand how peptides reduce inflammation, renew skin, and boost overall energy without causing strain or imbalance.
- **A new way to think about wellness:** Realize that peptides help your body remember how to function efficiently and naturally, rather than forcing change.

What Exactly Are Peptides?

Peptides are one of the body's most powerful communication tools, tiny yet incredibly influential. They function as messengers, carrying vital instructions that maintain system balance and proper function. Every bodily process, including healing, growth, metabolism, and inflammation control, depends on these molecules. Although they have always been part of your biology, modern understanding now allows us to use them intentionally to restore vitality, repair damage, and enhance performance.

Key Concepts

- **Definition:** Peptides are short chains of amino acids, the same components that make up proteins.
- **The difference between peptides and proteins:** Proteins are large and complex, whereas peptides are smaller and faster-acting.
- **How peptides work:** They send direct messages to specific receptors in your cells, prompting clear biological responses like healing, energy production, or growth.
- **Examples of natural peptide activity:**
    - Growth hormone release
    - Appetite regulation
    - Anti-inflammatory signaling
    - Tissue and wound repair
- **Why peptides matter now:** Modern science has learned to harness and support these natural signals to guide the body's repair and renewal processes more effectively.

The Signal Problem After 35

As we pass our mid-thirties, subtle yet powerful shifts occur as our effortlessly communicating systems begin to **slow down**. Cellular messages weaken, recovery takes longer, and energy levels decline. While this is a natural part of aging , modern life (stress, poor sleep, constant stimulation) exacerbates this slowdown. The good news is that the body still knows how to function optimally; it simply needs help **turning the volume back up** on its internal signals.

Key Insights

- **Weaker cellular communication:** Aging reduces the efficiency of cell-to-cell signaling, resulting in less clarity of internal messages for growth, repair, and energy.
- **Reduced receptor activity:** Fewer receptors are expressed on cells, making it more difficult for vital messages (such as those for healing or fat metabolism) to be transmitted.
- **Rising oxidative stress:** Over time, increased oxidative stress damages cells and further disrupts cellular communication.
- **Lifestyle disruptions:** Poor sleep, high stress, and artificial light interfere with the circadian rhythm and hormone balance.
- **Visible effects:**
  - Decrease in nighttime growth hormone production
  - Slower collagen renewal
  - Reduced fat burning
  - Longer recovery after workouts or injuries
- **How traditional fixes miss the mark:** Common solutions like stimulants, extreme diets, or excessive training mask the problem by pushing the body harder instead of repairing the root cause.
- **The peptide solution:** Peptides restore clear communication by **amplifying the body's natural signals**, helping the system operate efficiently without stress or exhaustion.

Peptides vs. Hormones vs. Supplements (Plain-English Comparison)

Understanding the difference between peptides, hormones, and supplements is key to making smarter health choices. Hormones are **powerful, system-wide messengers**; supplements provide **nutritional support**; and peptides deliver **precise instructions** that guide the body toward balance and repair. Knowing their distinct roles provides clarity on which approach to combine or choose for personal wellness goals.

Key Comparisons:

Category	Role	Function & Impact
Peptides	Targeted Messengers	Activate existing pathways quickly and precisely. Improve repair, fat metabolism, collagen production, immune function, and sleep quality. Help the body correct imbalances gently.
Hormones	Powerful, System-Wide Messengers	Influence multiple organs and tissues at once. Beneficial for deficiencies, but require careful monitoring due to broad impact and potential side effects.
Supplements	Nutritional Building Blocks	Provide vitamins, minerals, and amino acids. Support overall health but typically lack the speed or precision for specific biological changes. Best used as a foundation, not a targeted corrective tool.

Why Precision Matters

Lasting health is about doing what's right for your body at the right time. Precise signals ensure the body responds efficiently and without unnecessary stress. Broad approaches like caffeine or stimulants provide temporary energy but often lead to burnout, poor sleep, and hormonal imbalance. Precision allows the body to work smarter, not harder, by sending targeted instructions that align with natural rhythms, restoring balance and performance without overwhelming the system.

Key Insights

- **Precision reduces stress:** Clear, accurate signals minimize strain on the body, preventing the side effects that result from overstimulation.

- **The problem with broadcasting:** Broad signals (e.g., stimulants) cause temporary energy but often lead to fatigue, disrupted sleep, and slower fat loss over time.
- **What precise signaling looks like:**
  - Encouraging natural, nighttime growth hormone release.
  - Boosting collagen production exactly where the skin needs repair.
  - Mobilizing stored fat for energy within specific time windows.

Peptides work with the body by supporting its existing communication pattern.

Core Categories You'll Use in This Book

This guide is structured to be results-driven and simple, organized by what you actually want to achieve. It includes clear "Starter Stacks" and timelines to help you track progress and make informed adjustments. The goal is clarity, providing a structured path to better health.

Main Peptide Categories

- **Metabolic & Fat Loss:** Focuses on improving metabolism, mobilizing stored fat, and increasing energy efficiency.
  - Examples: CJC-1295 + Ipamorelin, AOD-9604
- **Muscle & Recovery:** Designed to boost growth hormone release, enhance muscle repair, and speed recovery after exercise or injury.
  - Examples: CJC-1295 + Ipamorelin, BPC-157, TB-500
- **Joints & Soft-Tissue Repair:** Targets inflammation, connective tissue repair, and joint regeneration for improved mobility and resilience.
  - Examples: BPC-157, TB-500, GHK-Cu
- **Skin, Hair & Beauty:** Promotes collagen production, cellular renewal, and healthy hair and skin appearance.
  - Examples: GHK-Cu, PTD-DBM combinations, Epitalon
- **Sleep, Energy & Mood:** Supports natural circadian rhythm, boosts cellular energy, and stabilizes mood for balanced well-being.
  - Examples: DSIP, Epitalon protocols

- **Gut & Immunity:** Strengthens gut lining integrity and enhances immune balance for better digestion and resilience.
    - Examples: BPC-157 for gut repair, Thymosin Alpha-1 for immune support
- **Longevity & Mitochondria:** Aims to improve cellular energy production, slow aging processes, and support long-term vitality.
    - Examples: Epitalon, MOTS-C

Each section provides step-by-step guidance on starter stacks, expected outcomes, and practical timelines to help you achieve your goals.

How Peptides Actually Work (Without Jargon)

Peptides are your body's **communication specialists**. They deliver clear, specific messages that tell cells exactly what to do, restoring order where signals have become quiet. They work by activating the right processes at the right time, without overpowering the system or causing unnecessary stimulation. Once their job is done, the body naturally breaks them down and clears them, making them efficient and gentle.

Key Concepts

- **The key-and-lock concept:** Each peptide connects with a matching **receptor** on the cell surface, like a key fitting perfectly into a lock.
- **What happens next:** Binding triggers a specific series of intracellular actions:
    - Enzymes are activated
    - Genes are switched on
    - Proteins are created or regulated
- **Why specificity matters:** Because each receptor only responds to its matching peptide, different peptides can act in the same body area to produce very different results (e.g., one signals growth hormone release, another boosts collagen).
- **Fast, focused, and efficient:** Peptides are small and precise, so they work quickly and are rapidly cleared from the body after delivering their message.

- **Safety through design:** This "quick on, quick off" nature helps prevent overstimulation and contributes to peptides being well-tolerated when used appropriately.

Safety Essentials You'll Learn in This Book

Using peptides safely is a core principle. Following proper practices ensures an effective response without unwanted side effects. The book emphasizes precision and consistency as the foundation of both safety and success.

Key Safety Concepts

- **Sourcing:** Learn to identify legitimate labs and recognize red flags to ensure product quality and safety.
- **Reconstitution & Storage:** Understand how to properly mix, label, and store peptides to maintain stability and effectiveness.
- **Dosing & Frequency:** Learn that more is not always better and how to optimize dose and timing for your goals and achieve optimal results.
- **Cycling & Pausing:** Explore strategies to prevent the body from adapting and to manage fatigue, timing stacks for maximum benefit without overuse.
- **Injection Site Rotation:** Learn proper rotation techniques to maintain healthy skin and ensure consistent absorption.

What Results Feel Like (Realistic Timelines)

When peptide protocols are combined with proper sleep, nutrition, and recovery, many people notice changes quickly. Peptides reactivate natural signaling pathways, which often respond fast to support metabolism, repair, and wellness. Realistic timelines help set expectations and maintain motivation.

Typical Progression

- **Weeks 1–2:** Experience **deeper, more restorative sleep**, less morning stiffness, and improved appetite control.
- **Weeks 3–4:** Notice visible reductions in stubborn fat areas, **brighter skin**, and better performance in workouts.

- **Weeks 6–8:** Muscle fullness and strength become more apparent, mobility improves, and post-workout recovery speeds up.
- **Weeks 10–12:** Friends may start noticing changes; you will feel lighter, clearer, more resilient, and energized.

Progress is measurable and trackable, which is supported by the program's journal, stack guide, and meal plan.

Mini Case Story: "I Didn't Change My Life, Just My Signals"

Jared, 44, who was dedicated to fitness but felt soft, sore, and wired at night , tried a conservative growth hormone-supporting stack: **CJC-1295 plus Ipamorelin** at bedtime. Within three weeks, he saw no drastic transformation, but found **consistency**: he was asleep by 10:30 p.m., experienced fewer aches, had more vigorous workouts, and a leaner waistline. This story highlights that the most powerful changes come from **supporting the body's own communication system**, allowing its natural rhythms to function effectively.

The Power Wellness Lens

This book employs a straightforward, practical framework, a roadmap for working *with* your body, not against it. Following these four phases helps restore communication, reinforce progress, and maintain results.

The Four Phases

- **Signal:** Use peptides to re-establish **clear, precise messages** between cells.
- **Support: Eat, move, and recover** in ways that reinforce those signals.
- **Stack: Combine complementary peptides** and protocols to achieve a single goal, maximizing efficiency.
- **Sustain:** Preserve your gains through **intelligent cycling**, consistent habits, and long-term lifestyle strategies.

By thinking in terms of signals and guiding your body with clarity, wellness becomes a natural and achievable conversation, not a struggle.

Your Starter Map (What To Do First)

To get started, focus on your main goal and follow a conservative, proven approach. This map guides focus; begin simply and track your progress to see results without overwhelming yourself.

Starter Approaches by Goal

Goal	Consideration	Why
Fat Loss + Better Sleep	CJC-1295 (no DAC) + Ipamorelin at bedtime; AOD-9604 in the morning	Nighttime GH pulses support recovery/fat mobilization; daytime AOD-9604 promotes fat breakdown
Muscle Rebuild + Joint Comfort	CJC-1295 + Ipamorelin for recovery; BPC-157 for soft-tissue support	GH pulses enhance muscle repair; BPC-157 supports tendon and ligament healing
Skin Glow + Hair Vitality	GHK-Cu topical (± systemic options with guidance) ± PTD-DBM blends	Stimulates collagen remodeling and hair follicle signaling
Gut Calm + Immunity Support	BPC-157 for gut lining; Thymosin Alpha-1 for immune tone (with clinical oversight)	Restores gut barrier function and balances immune signaling

These guidelines serve as a framework for understanding expected progress, rather than medical prescriptions.

Sample Peptide Stack

Attribute	Detail
Name	Fat-Loss Accelerator
Peptides	CJC-1295 (no DAC) + Ipamorelin; AOD-9604
Primary Goal	Boost nighttime GH pulses and trigger fat mobilization during the day
Suggested Timing	CJC-1295 + Ipamorelin at bedtime; AOD-9604 first thing in the morning
Cycle	8–12 weeks, then reassess
Tips for Success	Pair AOD-9604 with a higher-protein breakfast; finish last meal 3 hours before bed; track progress in your Journal

This stack supports natural signaling for safe and effective fat loss, as well as optimized sleep patterns, when combined with proper nutrition and recovery.

Myths You Can Let Go Of

Understanding the truth about common peptide misconceptions helps you approach their use with confidence and effectiveness.

Myth	Reality
Myth 1: "Peptides are steroids."	Reality: Steroids are hormones with broad systemic effects. Peptides are short chains of amino acids that act locally, aligning with your physiology and avoiding steroid-like side effects
Myth 2: "If a little works, a lot works better."	Reality: Precision signaling is not improved by overdosing; more can lead to chaos. Timing, rhythm, and sleep are the actual multipliers

Myth 3: "Once I stop, everything goes away."	Reality: Supportive habits (such as sleep, protein, and resistance training) maintain their benefits. Peptides rebuild capacity; your habits preserve it
Myth 4: "It's too complicated."	Reality: The process is manageable by focusing on one goal and one stack at a time, using the Journal to simplify tracking key metrics

Peptides are a tool for supporting natural intelligence, not a shortcut, gimmick, or source of stress.

Metrics That Matter (What You'll Track)

Tracking the right metrics helps you measure real progress without relying on guesswork. Focusing on key areas provides a clear view of how your body responds to peptides, nutrition, and recovery.

Key Metrics to Track

- **Sleep:** Record time to fall asleep, nighttime awakenings, and morning energy levels (1–10 scale).
- **Body Composition:** Track waist measurements, take progress photos, and log strength reps at consistent weights.
- **Recovery:** Note delayed onset muscle soreness (1–10 scale) and monitor joint comfort during daily activity.
- **Skin & Hair:** Observe skin texture, brightness, and hair shedding weekly to track improvements.
- **Digestion:** Track bloating, bowel regularity, and post-meal comfort to monitor gut response.

Logging these simple metrics daily provides significant insights and allows for adjustments to the approach by the end of the first month.

Nutrition Without Confusion (Why the Meal Plan Works)

Peptides amplify signals, but they cannot replace a balanced nutrition strategy. When meals support these signals, results are stronger, faster, and more sustainable.

The **30-Day Power Meal Plan** is designed to maintain high protein levels, balance carbohydrates with physical activity, and provide recovery-focused nutrients timed to support restful sleep. It is practical, flexible, and avoids extreme restrictions.

Sample Meal Plan Day

- **Breakfast:** Greek yogurt protein bowl with berries and chia seeds (protein-forward)
- **Lunch:** Grilled chicken power salad with olive oil vinaigrette
- **Snack:** Cottage cheese with pineapple
- **Dinner:** Salmon with roasted asparagus and quinoa
- **Evening:** Herbal tea; kitchen closed **3 hours before bed**

This simple, nourishing, and well-timed plan supports peptide signaling, optimizes recovery, and makes the wellness journey achievable.

Sleep: The Non-Negotiable Multiplier

Sleep is the **ultimate performance enhancer** for any peptide protocol. Nighttime is when the body repairs, rebuilds, and resets: growth hormone pulses occur, collagen synthesis takes place, and the brain clears toxins. Even the best-designed stack delivers limited results if sleep is inconsistent.

Sleep Optimization Tips

- Maintain a **consistent bedtime and wake-up time**.
- Keep your room **dark and cool**.
- Avoid **heavy meals** close to bedtime.
- Minimize **screen exposure** before lights-out.

Prioritizing sleep amplifies the effects of your peptide stack and makes all other efforts (nutrition, training, supplementation) more effective and sustainable.

What About GLP-1 Medications?

Peptides can be used in conjunction with GLP-1 medications (such as Semaglutide or Tirzepatide), which are often employed for appetite management and weight loss. Peptides help preserve lean muscle, support deeper sleep, and accelerate recovery, even when calorie intake is reduced. This book offers clear guidance on the compatibility of peptides and GLP-1 medications, highlighting situations where overlapping signals should be avoided.

Ethics, Legality, and Working With Professionals

The regulatory landscape for peptides is rapidly evolving, making it crucial to understand the rules and guidelines for safe and responsible use.

Key Principles

- **Work with qualified professionals:** Discuss peptide options with a **licensed clinician** who can provide guidance tailored to your health profile.
- **Follow current regulations:** Stay informed about legal guidelines to ensure responsible use of your resources.
- **Make conservative, informed choices:** Prioritize safety and alignment with your goals over chasing aggressive protocols.

Empowerment comes through knowledge combined with careful execution and professional oversight, maximizing benefits while minimizing risk.

Your Mindset Moving Forward

View peptides as a tool for **precise communication**, not a shortcut or a thrill ride. Approach the process with **curiosity, consistency, and attention to detail**. Track your progress and make minor adjustments to see how quickly your body responds to clear signals. The goal is to restore your body's natural design and function, not chase hacks.

Now that you understand what peptides are and why they matter, the next step is learning how they interact with your cells. In Chapter 2, you'll meet the **receptors, the** microscopic locks that make peptides safe, specific, and effective when used with rhythm and respect. You will also find an **at-a-glance chart** of the top clinically studied peptides and their functions.

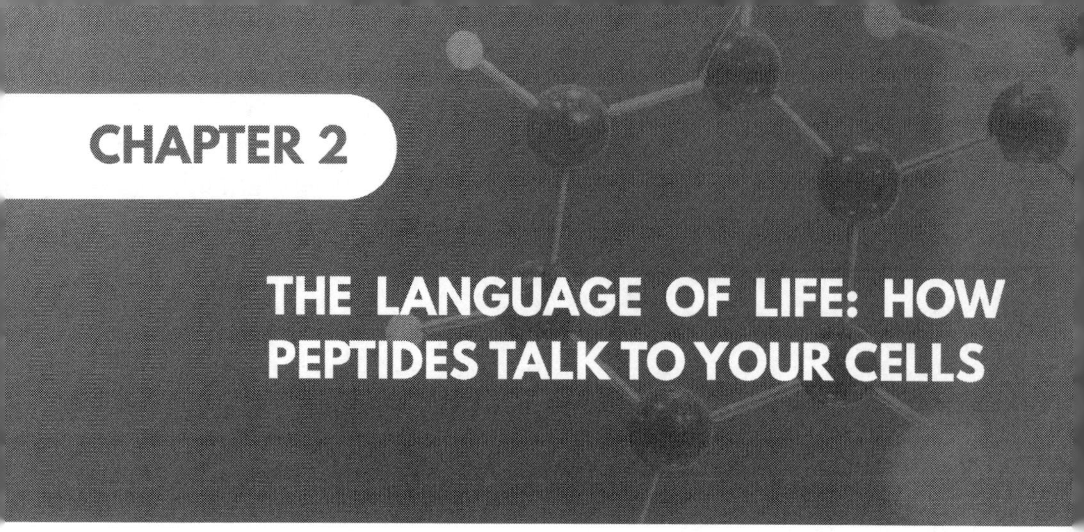

CHAPTER 2

THE LANGUAGE OF LIFE: HOW PEPTIDES TALK TO YOUR CELLS

As a child, your body seemed to heal effortlessly. Scrapes mended quickly, colds vanished without medication, and you awoke with energy, even after little sleep. This wasn't merely good luck; it was your body communicating with perfect clarity. Every act of repair, adjustment, and vitality stemmed from your cells being perfectly in sync, sending precise instructions on what to do and when to do it.

This chapter details how this vital internal communication occurs, why it naturally degrades over time, and how peptides can help restore it systematically. Understanding this biological process will provide you with the necessary clarity and confidence to use peptides safely and effectively, grounded in how your body truly operates.

The Conversation Within

Your body is a vibrant, living **communication network**. Every second, trillions of cells are engaged in sending, receiving, and responding to chemical signals that maintain your life and overall balance. This continuous, hidden dialogue governs everything you experience, from how fast you recover and how deeply you sleep to your daily energy levels. When this communication is fluid, you feel strong and energetic. When it falters, your body begins to struggle to keep up. Grasping this internal language is the critical first step toward accessing your body's inherent intelligence and rejuvenating its youthful rhythm.

Key Ideas:

- Your body is composed of **trillions of cells** that work collaboratively for survival, communication, and maintaining balance.
- Cells do not use spoken words; instead, they communicate via **chemical signals**, a process known as **cellular communication**.
- Every essential function you rely on, including metabolism, healing, immunity, energy, mood, and sleep, depends on this **clear, targeted cellular communication**.
- **Hormones** function like **public announcements** to the entire body: they are broad, powerful, and often less precise in their effects.
- **Peptides** act more like **private messages**: they are short, specific, and directed only to precise targets within the body.
- When a peptide reaches its corresponding **receptor** (which acts like a mailbox on the cell's surface), it delivers a clear, specific instruction.
- The cell immediately responds by undertaking a task such as repairing tissue, reducing inflammation, generating growth factors, or boosting energy utilization.
- This microscopic exchange happens millions of times every second, driving your body's adaptation, recovery, and renewal processes.
- **Strong peptide signaling** keeps your body in perfect harmony, like a well-conducted orchestra.
- **Weak signaling** is directly linked to negative outcomes such as a slower metabolism, chronic fatigue, increased inflammation, and accelerated aging.
- Peptides help restore this clarity, **reigniting the internal conversation** that is essential for health, energy, and resilience.
- Strengthening this communication is fundamentally about **activating the blueprint of vitality** that has always existed within you.

When the Signal Starts to Fade

As we progress through adulthood, the body's sophisticated communication system naturally begins to **decelerate**. Around the **mid-thirties**, many individuals start noticing subtle shifts: decreased energy, slower recovery from activity, and weight that is harder to manage. This is not simply about age; it's a clear indication that your cells are not "hearing" each other as clearly as they once did.

Furthermore, the demands of modern life introduce significant **noise** into this vital system. Factors like chronic stress, poor sleep patterns, rapid sugar fluctuations, and exposure to environmental toxins all interfere with the chemical messages your cells rely on for optimal function. The result is a body operating through a state of **static,** it's still working, but never at its full, youthful capacity. Recognizing this gradual decline is the first essential step toward reestablishing clear and youthful cellular communication, which helps your body recover its energy, balance, and overall vitality.

Key Ideas:

- Around the age of **35**, cell receptors naturally become **less sensitive** to the signals that regulate essential functions like fat burning, tissue repair, and recovery.
- **Daily stressors** exacerbate this problem by disrupting the body's internal chemical messaging system.
- The primary factors that **disrupt cellular communication** are:
    - **Chronic stress**
    - **Blood sugar imbalances**
    - **Poor or inconsistent sleep**
    - **Ongoing inflammation**
    - **Environmental toxins**
- These factors generate "**static**" within your internal communication system, akin to attempting to send an important message over a weak internet connection.
- When essential signals are missed or significantly delayed, the consequences can manifest as:
    - **Constant tiredness** or persistently low energy
    - **Slower healing** following injuries or workouts

    - Stubborn body fat, particularly around the midsection
    - Dull or thinning skin
    - Brain fog and unpredictable energy levels
- This biological slowdown is not a sign of failure but is the body's **feedback**, a request from your cells for clearer instructions.
- Peptides are instrumental in **strengthening that cellular connection**, enabling your system to transmit and receive messages with greater efficiency.
- As signaling is optimized, metabolism is **reawakened**, repair processes accelerate, and vitality naturally returns from within.

Here's what's really happening:

System Decline	What Declines	What You Feel
Growth-Hormone Axis	Fewer nighttime pulses of growth hormone	Increased fat storage and slower recovery after activity
Collagen Signaling	Reduced fibroblast activity, limiting collagen production	Wrinkles, sagging skin, and stiffness in the joints
Mitochondrial Signals	Lower cellular energy output	Midday fatigue and reduced stamina
Immune Communication	Imbalance in cytokine signaling	More inflammation and slower healing or repair

Mitochondrial Function: Mitochondria are the power plants within your cells that convert food and oxygen into usable energy (ATP). When they slow down, you experience tiredness, prolonged recovery, and fewer calories burned. Specific peptides are specifically designed to enhance **mitochondrial efficiency**, helping cells produce energy more effectively and cleanly.

Cytokine Signaling: This refers to the sophisticated way your **immune cells** communicate using small protein messengers called **cytokines**. These messengers instruct cells on when to activate, repair, or calm down inflammation, enabling your body to fight infection, heal injuries, and maintain overall balance. Clear, balanced cytokine signaling ensures your immune system operates as a unified, coordinated team. Conversely, an overactive or sluggish state can result in chronic inflammation, fatigue, prolonged recovery, or autoimmune conditions.

Peptides function like a **router upgrade**. They don't change the content of the body's messages; they simply boost the signal strength so that all internal instructions are delivered clearly and effectively.

The Lock-and-Key Model

Within your body, every peptide has an exact, specific destination; this is **precision biology** in action, not randomness. Each peptide actively searches for and finds a **matching receptor** on a cell's surface, analogous to a perfectly shaped **key finding its lock**.

The instant this connection is established, it initiates a **chain reaction** inside the cell. This reaction can activate enzymes, switch on specific genes, synthesize new proteins, or trigger the release of hormones. This mechanism allows your body to respond with exceptional **accuracy and balance**, rather than being overwhelmed.

Key Ideas:

- Each peptide is structured to fit only **one specific type of receptor**, guaranteeing targeted communication.
- The binding of a peptide to its receptor triggers an immediate and **precise cellular response**.
- These critical responses include **tissue repair**, the release of hormones, or the **synthesis of proteins**.
- Because peptides act locally and with high specificity, they are generally considered **safer and gentler** than drugs that saturate the entire system.
- Their precision helps the body **restore its natural rhythms** instead of forcefully overriding them.

Example in Action: The peptide *CJC-1295* specifically targets receptors in the pituitary gland to cue a natural growth hormone pulse. Rather than forcing non-stop hormone production, it helps to reestablish your body's original, healthy rhythm, particularly the essential nighttime surge that drives deep recovery and repair during sleep.

Peptides fundamentally work with your biology, not against it. By fitting into specific receptors, they deliver precise messages that help your body intelligently and naturally restore balance, vitality, and youthful function.

A Brief Tour of Cellular Messaging

Your body is involved in a continuous internal dialogue. Millions of peptide signals flash across your cells every second, orchestrating essential functions like growth, repair, energy, and balance. This is an elegant biological language that preserves your youthful state, strength, and adaptability. When this communication is clear, your body knows exactly when to build, when to rest, and when to heal.

Here is the four-step process of cellular communication:

- **Signal Release:** A gland, specific tissue, or a peptide supplement releases a messenger molecule into the bloodstream or surrounding tissue. This is either a natural part of the body's repair instructions or an amplified signal provided by therapeutic peptides.
- **Travel:** The peptide navigates through the bloodstream or tissue fluid, carrying its precise message. It coordinates complex systems, such as metabolism, recovery, and immunity, by directing signals to the cells that most need them, often within seconds.
- **Binding:** Upon locating its matching receptor, the peptide briefly connects, acting as a key in a lock. This binding moment **activates the signal**, immediately sparking cellular action.
- **Response:** The cell executes tasks such as repairing tissue, lowering inflammation, generating collagen, or burning stored fat. The positive physical benefits you observe, like improved energy, smoother skin, and quicker healing, all originate at this microscopic level.

- **Clearance:** After its message is fully delivered, the peptide is rapidly broken down and removed by enzymes. This **short life cycle** is essential for preventing overstimulation and maintaining a responsive and balanced system.

Peptide signaling works in seamless harmony with your body's inherent intelligence and timing. Every signal knows when to begin and when to stop, maintaining the precise cellular communication necessary for an efficient and balanced body, free from overwhelm. This natural rhythm of sending the message, performing the task, and then resetting makes peptide communication one of the most remarkable systems for continuous repair and renewal.

Precision vs. Force

For many years, various health interventions have depended on **force** rather than biological finesse. The philosophy was straightforward: push harder by adding more hormones, more stimulants, or more severe restrictions. While these methods can yield rapid, superficial results, they often come at a significant cost: the body becomes overstressed, develops dependency, or ultimately suffers burnout from being pushed beyond its natural limits.

Precision signaling operates on a completely different premise. Instead of forcing a change, it subtly and gently **activates the body's existing pathways**. It serves as a reminder to your system of *what to do*, rather than attempting to replace a missing component. This balanced approach encourages **homeostasis**, allowing the body to naturally restore its own rhythm and strength instead of causing overload.

Peptides perfectly embody this principle by acting as highly precise messengers, guiding the body to respond intelligently and efficiently. When people describe the effects of peptides as feeling "**natural**," it is because they are entirely aligned with the body's innate design. They do not override or replace hormones; they encourage your system to naturally produce and regulate, restoring critical timing and balance within your biology.

Synergy: Why Some Peptides Work Better Together

Peptides achieve their maximum effectiveness when they **complement one another**. Just like individual instruments in an orchestra, certain combinations significantly enhance the body's natural processes far more than any single peptide could alone. This is the foundational reason why strategic pairing, often called **stacking**, is used in the Power Wellness system.

Examples of Effective Peptide Synergy:

- **CJC-1295 + Ipamorelin:** CJC-1295 stimulates the release of growth hormone, while Ipamorelin amplifies the pulses. Together, they successfully mimic the body's natural nighttime rhythms, profoundly supporting regeneration and recovery.
- **BPC-157 + TB-500:** BPC-157 concentrates on repairing local tissue damage, and TB-500 enhances blood flow to deliver nutrients and oxygen faster. The combination dramatically accelerates overall healing and tissue restoration.
- **GHK-Cu + Epitalon:** GHK-Cu promotes the production of collagen, and Epitalon supports cellular longevity. Their combined action works to enhance skin health, vitality, and overall rejuvenation.

In nature, very few biological systems function in total isolation. Stacking is fundamentally about **collaboration** and achieving a greater effect, not about unnecessarily adding complexity.

Top 10 Clinically Studied Peptides at a Glance

Peptide	Primary Function	Common Outcome
CJC-1295 / Ipamorelin	Stimulates growth-hormone pulses	Supports fat loss and faster recovery
AOD-9604	Enhances fat metabolism	Targeted fat reduction
BPC-157	Promotes tissue repair	Speeds up injury recovery
TB-500 (Thymosin Beta-4)	Improves blood flow and healing	Relieves joint and tendon issues
GHK-Cu	Collagen and hair support	Skin rejuvenation and hair health
Epitalon	Supports telomeres	Promotes longevity and better sleep
MOTS-C	Boosts mitochondrial energy	Enhances metabolic health
Thymosin Alpha-1	Modulates immune function	Fewer infections and improved defense
DSIP	Sleep-inducing peptide	"Deeper, more restorative rest"
LL-37	Antimicrobial peptide	Supports gut and immune health

Telomere: Telomeres are like the protective plastic tips on shoelaces, capping the ends of your chromosomes. They shorten each time a cell divides, and when they become too short, the cell ages or dies because it can no longer divide properly. Certain peptides, such as Epitalon, are believed to help maintain the length of telomeres, supporting healthier cellular aging and longevity.

Immune Modulation: Modulation means **balancing** the immune system, not just forcefully boosting it. Peptides that modulate help your body respond appropriately, avoiding both overreaction with inflammation and under-reaction to an infection. The primary goal is **homeostasis,** restoring balance in immune communication so that healing can occur without excessive, damaging inflammation.

Sleep Induction: Certain peptides, such as **DSIP** (Delta Sleep-Inducing Peptide), interact directly with your natural **circadian rhythm** to facilitate your body's entry into deeper, more restorative sleep phases. They do not sedate you like traditional sleeping pills; instead, they signal the body to initiate its natural biological processes of rest and recovery.

Antimicrobial Peptides: These are small, protein-like molecules that your body produces naturally to defend against fungi, viruses, and bacteria. They are a crucial component of your innate immune system, serving as the first line of defense before antibodies are deployed. Some synthetic or enhanced peptides are designed to mimic the action of these natural defenders.

Microinflammation: Also known as **low-grade chronic inflammation**, this is a silent, slow type of inflammation that occurs at the cellular level. It is often triggered by aging, stress, processed foods, or toxins. Unlike injury pain, it does not hurt, but its long-term effect is to erode cellular communication and repair mechanisms. Specific peptides can help to quiet these low-grade inflammatory signals, promoting better regeneration.

Educational disclaimer: *Research into these peptides is still in its preliminary stages, and human results may vary significantly. You must always consult a licensed medical professional before beginning any new use or protocol.*

The Language Analogy

Imagine your body as a dynamic, complex city. Every system has a designated role, and constant communication is what keeps everything running smoothly.

- **Hormones** are like the **mayor's public announcements**: they are broad, powerful, and intended for everyone in the city at once. An example would be: "Citywide curfew tonight!".
- **Supplements** are the **building materials** delivered to construction sites: they are certainly helpful, but they do not contain the instructions on how to actually use them.
- **Peptides** are the **emails sent between department heads**: they are timely, specific, and actionable instructions.

When these specific emails (peptides) are delayed or stop arriving, the city begins to struggle: trash piles up (inflammation), streetlights fail (mitochondrial fatigue), and necessary repairs lag behind (joint pain).

How Peptides Influence Major Systems

Peptides act as **master communicators**, sending precise instructions that effectively coordinate multiple major systems in your body. Each signal is designed to help maintain balance, repair damage, and optimize overall performance. Think of this as one unified language that coordinates every "neighborhood" of your body.

Major Systems Affected by Peptides:

- **Metabolic System:** They signal fat cells to release stored energy instead of hoarding it, thereby supporting overall energy balance and weight management.
- **Musculoskeletal System:** They direct muscle fibers to repair, grow, and strengthen in response to stress or injury.
- **Immune System:** They work to reduce excessive inflammation while simultaneously strengthening your body's natural defenses.
- **Neural System:** They are key to supporting mental clarity, mood stability, and healthy, restorative sleep cycles.

- **Dermal System:** They stimulate essential fibroblasts to produce collagen and elastin, which greatly improves skin elasticity and texture.
- **Digestive System:** They help restore the crucial integrity of the gut lining and balance the microbiome, leading to better overall digestion and immunity.

Although each system is complex, peptides communicate using a unified language that coordinates their functions to achieve optimal results. While future chapters will offer detailed protocols for each system, it is important to recognize now how a single, targeted signal can enhance the performance, resilience, and renewal of the entire body.

Why Age Isn't the Villain, Silence Is

We frequently assign blame to aging for common complaints like fatigue, slow recovery times, and weight gain that is resistant to change. However, a large part of this decline is actually due to **weakened cellular communication**, rather than just the passage of years. When this vital signaling is restored, the body is able to function much closer to its younger self. This principle explains why a 50-year-old who actively optimizes their peptide signaling can sometimes achieve better performance than a 30-year-old who is constantly running on stress and caffeine.

Peptides do not possess the ability to reverse age literally. Instead, they restore the essential **clarity of the messages** that your cells require to operate efficiently. By effectively turning the volume back up on cellular communication, they empower your body to perform, adapt, and recover as if it were decades younger.

A Day in the Life of Cellular Messaging

Your body functions like a perfectly tuned orchestra, with every system playing its part at the precise moment. Peptides act as the **conductors**, ensuring that every section remains in harmony throughout the day and night.

Daily Peptide Flow:

- **Morning: AOD-9604** signals fat cells to release stored energy, providing fuel for your day.
- **Afternoon: BPC-157** targets and addresses micro-inflammation caused by physical activity, thereby supporting tissue health and recovery.
- **Evening: CJC-1295 + Ipamorelin** triggers restorative growth-hormone pulses, aligning with your body's natural repair cycle as you begin to fall asleep.
- **Night: Epitalon** works to extend the deep-sleep cycles and support telomere maintenance, promoting crucial cellular longevity.

Epitalon (Epithalamin): This well-researched peptide, originally discovered in Russia, is known for its role in supporting telomere maintenance, providing antioxidant defense, and regulating sleep through its effect on **melatonin balance**. It is often associated with longevity research and is believed to function by optimizing the pineal gland and synchronizing the body's circadian rhythms.

When all these signals are clear and well-timed, your body operates with maximum efficiency and smoothness. Peptides act to fine-tune the entire system, correcting any "off-key" instruments so that every cell performs in sync, keeping you balanced, resilient, and energetic.

Why Men and Women Respond Differently

Men and women may experience distinct effects from the same peptide, not because the peptides change, but because of **biological variations** between the sexes.

- **Men** frequently observe quicker muscle repair, faster spikes in growth hormone, and more noticeable retention of lean muscle mass.
- **Women** often report stronger benefits related to fat metabolism, collagen production, improved sleep quality, and better mood regulation.

These differences in response are primarily driven by underlying factors such as varying **receptor density**, differing hormonal balances, and distinct enzyme activity. While the chemical language spoken by peptides is universal, the ultimate **timing, intensity, and duration** of the response is uniquely individual. Recognizing these innate biological differences allows for the development of tailored approaches. Future chapters will provide specific dosing ranges, cycle lengths, and timing windows optimized for both men and women to ensure safe and effective peptide results.

Supportive Habits That Magnify Results

Peptides are undeniably powerful tools, but their efficacy is largely contingent upon the **clarity of your body's communication channels**. Like any signal transmission, cellular messaging requires both energy and a well-maintained system to be fully effective. Therefore, supporting your peptide regimen with healthy lifestyle habits will dramatically amplify their benefits and enable your body to respond optimally.

Key Supportive Habits:

- **Protein:** Aim for a minimum of **0.8–1 gram of protein** per pound of lean body mass daily to provide the necessary building blocks for growth and repair.
- **Hydration:** Drink **80–100 ounces of water** daily, ensuring you include electrolytes, especially if you engage in intense training.
- **Sleep:** Consistently maintain a schedule that allows for **7–9 hours of sleep** per night to support signaling and recovery.
- **Movement:** Integrate a combination of **resistance training** with Zone-2 cardio to build strength, enhance endurance, and improve metabolic health.
- **Stress Management:** Actively practice breathwork, seek sunlight exposure, and cultivate gratitude to reduce the interference (static) in cellular communication.

These supportive habits are not merely optional extras; they are **essential amplifiers of our well-being**. A strong signal must pass through a clear and energized channel, making the restoration of calm, balanced cellular communication key to how peptides effectively work.

Mini Case Study: Sarah's Reset

Sarah, a 39-year-old manager of a demanding marketing team, was heavily reliant on coffee and was only averaging six hours of sleep per night. She began her protocol with **BPC-157** to specifically address chronic gut irritation, and later added the combined stack of **CJC-1295 + Ipamorelin** to be taken at night. Using the **30-Day Journal**, she consistently tracked her digestion, sleep quality, and daily energy levels.

- **Week 2:** She noticed a significant reduction in bloating.
- **Week 5:** She reported having "steady energy without needing caffeine".

By diligently documenting her progress, Sarah was able to identify real, measurable trends in her health, relying on data-driven results instead of mere hopeful speculation.

Sarah's Take: "It felt like my body finally got the memo".
Consistent tracking, when combined with the use of targeted peptides, allows you to clearly observe your body's response, transforming subtle initial improvements into truly measurable and lasting change.

How This Science Builds Trust

It is not necessary to memorize every chemical pathway or receptor to successfully benefit from peptides. What is truly essential is understanding that each peptide has a **specific target**, a clear purpose, and a **natural rhythm**.

Respecting that natural rhythm through proper cycling, adequate rest, and optimized nutrition is what makes outcomes reliable and predictable. This predictability is the fundamental reason why medical professionals, wellness coaches, and even Olympic recovery teams have increasingly integrated peptide protocols over the last decade.

Peptides deliver the best results when approached with knowledge and a deep respect for your body's natural rhythms. By faithfully following proven principles, you achieve safe and measurable results, fostering confidence in the underlying science.

Common Misfires (and How to Avoid Them)

Even the most targeted peptide protocols can fail to achieve their full potential if foundational principles are overlooked. Avoiding these common mistakes is crucial for maximizing your full benefit and safely remaining on track.

Top 5 Misfires:

1. **Skipping Sleep:** Most peptides that promote growth and repair are at their most active during the night. Missing out on sleep can reduce your results by half.
2. **Ignoring Nutrition:** A protein intake that is too low or following extreme fasting protocols deprives your body of the essential building blocks it needs for growth and repair.
3. **Overlapping Signals:** Using too many growth-hormone-releasing peptides simultaneously creates **signal noise**. Always adhere to the specific stacking guidelines provided in later chapters.
4. **Impatience:** Peptides operate according to the pace of biology, meaning that real, lasting results will emerge over a period of **weeks**, not merely days.
5. **Sourcing Blindly:** Using unreliable suppliers introduces the risk of impurity and ineffective results. Chapter 11 will provide guidance on how to vet your sources safely.

Steering clear of these five common misfires can effectively double your results and ensure your motivation remains high.

Integration With Your Toolkit

As you progress through this program, you will notice helpful **power cues** designed to guide your practice:

- **Stack Combos:** These highlight the recommended, synergistic peptide combinations.
- **Meal Plan:** This guides the optimal timing of your peptide use relative to your food windows to support strong signaling.
- **Journal:** This encourages you to track key indicators like energy, recovery, and sleep, to monitor and confirm your progress.

These tools are not optional additions; they collectively form an **accountability system** that converts knowledge into real-world, measurable results. They are essential for helping you apply peptides both safely and effectively.

Looking Ahead

At this point, you have a solid understanding of how peptides communicate with your cells and why that precise messaging is so critically important for maintaining health, repair, and vitality.

In **Chapter 3**, you will learn how to apply this foundational knowledge to one of the most sought-after goals: **reigniting a metabolism** that has slowed down over the years. You will discover why simple calorie restriction often fails, how peptides can safely restart the fat-burning process without causing hormonal disruption, and how your integrated **Meal Plan** and **Journal** will work together to track measurable, real progress in a period of just 30 days.

Your body inherently knows the language of renewal. Peptides do not teach it a new language; they simply help your cells **remember the signals**, guiding metabolism, recovery, and energy back to their peak, youthful performance.

CHAPTER 3

THE FAT-LOSS RESET: WHY DIETS FAIL AND HOW PEPTIDES RESTART METABOLISM

You might be consistently tracking your meals, hitting your goals, and following popular "effortless" fat-loss trends. Yet, despite your best efforts, your progress has stalled or even reversed. This isn't a sign of personal failure; it's your body's natural survival mechanism at work. When your body perceives restriction or famine, it naturally conserves energy and resists further fat loss. The initial step toward lasting fat loss is understanding and working with this built-in biological response.

This chapter focuses on:

- **Your body's natural defense:** How the perception of famine or stress leads to metabolic adaptation and slows progress.
- **Why quick-fix diets fail:** The hidden rebound effect associated with crash diets and extreme eating plans.
- **The truth about fat-loss plateaus:** Recognizing them not as failure, but as signals from your body asking for metabolic balance.
- **Working with your biology:** Employing smart nutrition, movement, and recovery strategies to restore metabolic trust.
- **The sustainable path:** Reigniting metabolism with smarter, less punishing methods that support long-term success.

Why Traditional Dieting Backfires After 35

Aging doesn't suddenly "break" your metabolism; instead, it causes your metabolism to adapt based on the signals it receives. Years of chronic stress, poor sleep, inconsistent eating, and repeated rounds of restrictive dieting teach the body to become cautious with its energy reserves. What is often mislabeled as a "slow metabolism" is actually a highly trained survival system. When the body senses restriction, it lowers thyroid output, conserves energy, and shifts its priority from burning to storage. The good news is that you can effectively re-train these signals through nourishment, appropriate movement, and peptide support, rather than continued deprivation or punishment.

Key Reasons Traditional Dieting Fails After 35:

- **Chronic Stress:** High cortisol levels promote fat storage and accelerate the breakdown of valuable lean muscle.
- **Poor Sleep:** Inadequate sleep reduces growth hormone production, a crucial factor in metabolic repair.
- **Reduced Activity:** Less spontaneous daily movement means a lower overall calorie burn.
- **Repeated Calorie Cuts:** Each cycle of dieting teaches the body to conserve energy and store fat more efficiently upon reintroduction of food.
- **Hormonal Imbalance:** Disruptions in key hormones, such as thyroid, leptin, and ghrelin, can increase hunger and fatigue.
- **Muscle Loss:** Dieting without sufficient protein causes the body to burn muscle along with fat, which permanently lowers your daily energy needs.
- **Weekend Rebound:** Strict restriction followed by overeating sends confusing signals, causing the body to become highly efficient at storing fat.

The Reset Approach offers a better solution than another extreme diet. It focuses on re-establishing transparent and predictable communication with your metabolism. This is achieved by focusing on consistent protein intake, strategic meal timing, resistance and Zone 2 training, which involves moderate, steady-state exercise that improves fat metabolism and endurance, and using targeted peptide stacks that encourage fat release while protecting lean mass.

The Three Levers That Move Fat Loss

Before you begin using peptides, your metabolic foundation must be solid. Peptides are not a replacement for healthy habits; they are amplifiers. If your foundation is weak, peptides won't work effectively. These three levers dictate your body's response to any fat-loss approach, including peptide protocols.

1. **Protein Priority**
   - Aim for 0.8–1.0 grams of protein per pound of lean body mass.
   - Protein is essential for muscle preservation during a calorie deficit, promotes satiety, and aids in repair while you sleep.
   - Centering your meals around protein ensures you burn fat, not muscle, as you get leaner.
2. **Glycemic Control**
   - Choose fiber-rich carbohydrates like vegetables, legumes, and whole grains.
   - Time your carbs strategically around workouts or movement to boost insulin sensitivity.
   - Stable blood sugar prevents fat-storing signals from taking over your metabolism and reduces cravings.
3. **Sleep & Stress Management**
   - High levels of stress and poor sleep elevate cortisol, making fat loss significantly harder.
   - Prioritize consistency in your bedtime, and include calming routines like light stretching or breathwork.
   - Deep sleep is a natural ally for fat loss, as it stabilizes insulin response and restores crucial growth hormone rhythms.

By aligning these three levers first, nutrition, blood sugar, and recovery, peptides can reach their full potential. A strong foundation transforms peptide therapy from an unsure experiment into a reliable and measurable transformation.

Why Peptides Help Where Diets Stumble

Traditional dieting focuses primarily on what you eat, but peptides focus on how your cells respond to your efforts. Peptides work by improving cellular signaling, which helps with nutrient partitioning, moderating appetite cues, and supporting recovery during sleep. This mechanism allows you to maintain a manageable calorie deficit without extreme deprivation, encouraging your body to shift toward fat burning while protecting lean muscle.

Practical Benefits of Peptide Support:

- Significantly reduced feelings of intense hunger and cravings.
- Deeper, more restorative sleep that enhances metabolic repair.
- Targeted fat loss in difficult areas like the waist, belly, and hips, while preserving muscle definition in the shoulders and arms.

Peptides are not merely for shrinking your size; they help re-compose your body. The core goal is to optimize and reshape how your cells utilize energy, resulting in fat loss that is smoother, more sustainable, and aligned with your body's natural biological rhythms.

Meet the Fat-Loss Signaling Trio

While many peptides affect body composition, this trio is particularly effective and synergistic for initial cycles, working together to mobilize fat, preserve lean mass, and enhance recovery.

CJC-1295 (no DAC) + Ipamorelin (Night Protocol)

- Function: Stimulates the body's natural growth hormone (GH) pulses during early sleep. GH helps mobilize fat, preserve lean tissue, improve sleep quality, enhance recovery, and support collagen turnover.
- Timing: Dosed at night to align with your natural circadian rhythms and minimize grogginess.
- Expected Results: Smoother sleep within 1–2 weeks; noticeable improvements in the midsection by weeks 3–6 with consistent nutrition.

AOD-9604 (Morning Cue)

- Function: Delivers a gentle, non-stimulant signal to the adipose (fat) tissue, encouraging lipolysis (the use of stored fat).
- Timing: Dosed in the morning to capitalize on naturally lower insulin levels, reinforcing fat mobilization.
- Expected Results: Subtle appetite regulation and a noticeable tightening in stubborn areas after 2–4 weeks.

BPC-157 (Recovery Support During Training)

- Function: Accelerates soft-tissue recovery and reduces micro-inflammation, enabling more frequent and effective workouts.
- Importance for Fat Loss: Protecting muscle mass while dieting is critical because it increases your daily calorie burn and improves overall body composition.

This trio effectively tackles the three core components of fat loss: mobilizing stored fat, preserving muscle, and supporting recovery. When combined with consistent movement, sleep, and nutrition, these peptides establish a framework for lasting, measurable changes in body composition.

Starter Stacks (Conservative, Proven, Trackable)

Begin your journey by selecting one goal-aligned stack and diligently tracking your progress for 30 days. Avoid combining multiple stacks initially to ensure clarity and safety in tracking results.

- **Starter Stack A : "Sleep & Slim"**
  - Use When: You struggle with poor sleep and stubborn fat around the waist.
  - Peptides: CJC-1295 (no DAC) + Ipamorelin at bedtime; AOD-9604 in the morning.
  - Pair With: Meal Plan Weeks 1–2; a minimum of two resistance-training sessions plus two walks per week.
  - Expect: Better sleep by week 2; visible waistline changes between weeks 3–5.

- **Starter Stack B : "Train & Tighten"**
    - Use When: You are already consistent with lifting weights 2–3 times per week.
    - Peptides: Same as Stack A, but add BPC-157 during periods of higher-volume training.
    - Pair With: Meal Plan Weeks 1–4; focus on progressive overload in lifting; aim for 7,000–8,000 steps daily.
    - Expect: Improved muscle tone and retained strength within 4–6 weeks.
- **Starter Stack C : "Reboot & Recompose" (Gentle)**
    - Use When: You are recovering from illness, extended dieting, or general burnout.
    - Peptides: CJC-1295 + Ipamorelin at night only; delay adding AOD-9604 until your sleep has stabilized.
    - **Start with the Foundation Week (Metabolic Reset)** by incorporating clean, balanced meals to stabilize blood sugar, reduce inflammation, and prepare your body. **Then follow the structured Meal Plan for Weeks 1–3** to activate fat loss and muscle recovery. Include daily sunlight and short walks after meals to enhance progress.
    - Expect: Stable energy by week 2; gradual and steady fat reduction by weeks 4–6.

These stacks emphasize sleep, recovery, muscle preservation, and fat mobilization. When combined with tracking, consistent movement, and nutrition, they offer a clear, safe path to measurable body composition changes.

Timelines You Can Trust

Progress achieved with a structured Meal Plan and peptides is a steady process, not an overnight event. While you should expect minor fluctuations, consistent tracking will reveal a clear, positive overall trend.

Realistic Timeline for a Starter Stack:

- **Week 1:** Slight improvement in sleep, evening cravings begin to ease, but the scale may not yet show movement.

- **Week 2:** Morning energy feels more consistent, your waist feels looser, and post-training soreness fades more quickly.
- **Week 3:** Initial visible changes appear, clothing fits better, and the scale typically starts trending down by 0.5–1.0 lb per week.
- **Weeks 4–6:** Others begin to notice changes. You look tighter and more defined because of strong lean-mass retention, even if the total weight loss is modest.
- **Weeks 7–8:** This is a decision point: either continue the cycle for another four weeks or transition into a two-week maintenance break to protect your mood and thyroid function. Strategies for sustaining these results are covered in Chapter 13.

The Meal Plan Connection (How Food Supports Signals)

The 30-Day Power Meal Plan is not a restrictive crash diet. Its core purpose is to align your nutrition with the signals sent by your peptides, training, and recovery processes. By strategically timing carbohydrates around activity, prioritizing protein, and stopping meals three hours before bed, the plan supports growth hormone pulses, lean-mass preservation, and fat mobilization.

Macro & Timing Overview:

- **Weeks 1–2:** Focus on moderate calories, higher protein, and moderate carbs on training days; slightly lower carbs on rest days.
- **Weeks 3–4:** If compliance is high and energy remains steady, you may slightly reduce calories by 5–10%.
- **Fiber:** Aim for 25–35 g/day from sources like berries, greens, whole grains, and beans (as tolerated).
- **Hydration:** Drink 80–100 oz/day, incorporating electrolytes if you are training or sweating heavily.

A Sample Meal Day:

- **Breakfast (Protein-Forward):** Egg-white omelet with spinach and feta, plus berries.
- **Lunch:** Turkey and quinoa bowl with roasted vegetables and olive-oil vinaigrette.

- **Snack:** A protein shake with an apple.
- **Dinner:** Lean steak, a sweet potato, and arugula salad with lemon.
- **Wind-Down:** Chamomile tea; avoid consuming heavy snacks after dinner.

This Meal Plan is designed to enhance the biological messages your peptides are sending, supporting muscle preservation, fat loss, and recovery. When this synergy between nutrition, peptides, and movement is achieved, your results become trackable, predictable, and sustainable.

Training That Protects Your Metabolism

Training's purpose extends beyond simply burning calories; it is about sending the correct biological signal to your body. Smart training, when paired with peptides, signals your body to retain lean muscle, boost metabolic health, and efficiently release stored fat. The underlying goal is always sustainability, not physical exhaustion.

Core Training Framework:

- **Resistance Training:** Complete 2–3 sessions weekly that cover the five fundamental movement patterns: squat, hinge, push, pull, and carry. Keep your repetitions between 6–12 per set, making sure to leave 1–2 reps in reserve (RIR) to stimulate growth and repair without causing burnout.
- **Walking/Zone 2 Cardio:** Aim for 30–45 minutes on most days. This activity is crucial for building endurance and training your body to efficiently use fat for fuel without impeding muscle retention or recovery.
- **Intervals (Optional):** Include 6–10 short bursts of intensity once weekly, but only if your sleep and recovery are consistent. A small amount of intensity can boost fat mobilization, but too much can elevate cortisol and halt progress.

GLP-1 Users: How Peptides Fit

If you are currently using GLP-1 medications such as semaglutide or tirzepatide, peptides can provide vital support. While GLP-1s are effective for reducing appetite and promoting weight loss, they can also decrease energy levels and protein intake, which are factors that threaten your lean muscle mass and recovery. Peptides help to bridge this gap by strengthening the body's natural repair and regeneration pathways.

Practical Integration Tips:

- **Avoid Excessive Appetite Suppression:** The aim is balanced nourishment, not deeper restriction.
- **Use GH-Supporting Night Protocols:** Peptides like CJC-1295 + Ipamorelin help protect collagen, muscle, and sleep quality during calorie reduction.
- **Maintain High Protein Intake:** Even if your appetite is low, your body's need for protein for repair and recovery remains constant.
- **Manage Nausea:** If nausea occurs, switch to gentler meal textures, such as smoothies, soups, or soft proteins, and ensure you increase your electrolyte intake.

Plateaus: What They Mean and What to Do

A stall in progress is not a sign of failure; it typically signifies your body’s adaptation. Knowing how to interpret and respond to a plateau is key:

- **Audit Consistency:** Be honest about whether you are truly meeting your protein goals and closing the kitchen a few hours before bedtime. Small slips can accumulate.
- **Check Sleep:** If you are frequently waking up or engaging in late-night phone use, prioritize recovery. Poor sleep hinders fat loss more rapidly than missed workouts.
- **Nudge Movement:** Add a simple 1,500 steps per day or an extra 15-minute walk. Gradual, gentle increases are more effective than drastic changes.
- **Micro-Cut:** Slightly reduce your daily calories by 100–150 for a short period of 7–10 days (typically by reducing fats or starches), and then reassess your progress.

- **Refeed (Advanced):** If you experience low energy and a dip in mood, a single day with higher carbohydrates can help reset hormones and boost training drive. Only attempt this after 10–14 days of strong adherence to your deficit.
- **Strategic Maintenance:** If a plateau persists for three or more weeks despite strict adherence, switch to a maintenance phase for two weeks before restarting a gentle deficit. This protects your mindset, hormones, and thyroid.

Trouble-Shooting Fat-Loss Signals

Improving progress often involves understanding and responding to the messages your body sends, not just doing more. Low energy, cravings, or stubborn fat are not signs of failure; they are simply feedback. By learning to read these signals, you can make intelligent, minor adjustments that maintain progress without extreme restriction or burnout.

Quick Checks to Fine-Tune Your Rhythm:

- **Evening Cravings:** Increase fiber and protein at dinner for better satiety. Switch sugary desserts for protein yogurt and berries. If cleared by your clinician, consider magnesium glycinate at night to calm the nervous system.
- **Flat Workouts:** Mix 10–15 g of essential amino acids into your training drink and avoid cutting carbs on workout days. Your muscles require both energy and building blocks for recovery and performance.
- **Constipation:** Increase your daily fiber intake and incorporate kiwi or chia pudding. Ensure you hydrate earlier in the day and take a short walk after meals to aid digestion.
- **Poor Sleep (Even with Peptides):** Shift your caffeine intake earlier, ensure your room is dark, and keep your dinner on the lighter side. Maintain a consistent timing for your evening peptides and supplements.
- **Stubborn Belly Fat:** This is often the last area to lean out and the first to respond to stress. Before further calorie reduction, focus intensely on consistent sleep, balanced nutrition, and relaxation practices.

When symptoms appear or fat loss slows, your body is communicating with you, not betraying you. Strategic tweaks can restore balance, maintain a responsive metabolism, and help you move forward with greater confidence.

The Psychology of Steady Fat Loss

Fat loss success relies less on achieving perfection and more on consistency, adjustment, and showing up long enough for the progress to accumulate. View your efforts like steady deposits in a bank account, each quality night's sleep, balanced meal, and completed workout adds to your results. Setbacks are only temporary withdrawals, not a declaration of bankruptcy; the key is to keep investing daily.

Your Journal is your personal financial ledger for progress. Track daily metrics such as protein intake, sleep quality, step count, training performance, and how your clothes fit. Also, note emotional cues, cravings, and hunger levels. Within three weeks, you should notice steady energy, fewer cravings, and subtle physical changes, even if the scale is initially resistant.

Power Prompts for Reflection in your Journal:

- What action did I take today that made tomorrow's effort easier?
- Where did I encounter friction today, and how can I reduce it next time?
- Did I successfully protect my wind-down window before bed?
- What non-scale victory did I experience today (e.g., better mood, energy, clothing fit, strength)?

Sample Stack

- **Name:** Sleep & Slim, Starter A
- **Peptides:** CJC-1295 (no DAC) + Ipamorelin at bedtime; AOD-9604 in the morning
- **Cycle Duration:** 8–12 weeks, with a comprehensive progress check at week 8
- **Pair With:** Meal Plan Weeks 1–2, two resistance-training sessions weekly, and 7,000–8,000 daily steps

- **Tips for Best Results:**
  - Stop eating at least 3 hours before bed to support the natural release of Growth Hormone (GH).
  - Use your journal to track your morning energy and sleep quality throughout the week.
  - Avoid consuming caffeine after 2 p.m. to ensure consistent sleep and recovery.
  - Expect steadier sleep by week 2 and visible waistline changes by weeks 3–5 when combined with consistent meals and movement.

Safety, Sourcing, and Dosing Reminders

Safety is the paramount factor for your health and results. The focus should be on making clean, consistent progress, rather than rushing the outcome. Every decision should support confidence and longevity in the process.

Key Guidelines:

- **Purity Matters:** Refer to Chapter 11 for guidance on verifying trusted suppliers and avoiding contaminated or counterfeit products.
- **Sterility First:** Always maintain a clean technique and rotate injection sites. Use the provided injection map to prevent irritation or the development of scar tissue.
- **Dose Conservatively:** Start with the lowest effective dose, track your body's response, and only make adjustments under the guidance of a professional.
- **Cycle Intentionally:** Schedule mandatory rest periods between cycles. A well-rested system remains more responsive and adapts better over time.

Mini Story: From Scale Prison to Shape Freedom

Luis, aged 46, often let his mood be dictated by the number on the scale each morning. After three weeks on Starter Stack A and the Meal Plan, he shifted his focus from weight to waist and from stress to sleep. The results were surprising: his belt tightened by two notches, his mornings felt calmer and more energized, yet the scale had barely moved. "I stopped chasing a number and started building a body," he realized. His transformation was both mental and physical, proving that real progress is about gaining confidence and consistency, not just rapid weight loss.

When to Stop, Switch, or Sustain

- **Stop:** If you notice any unusual or uncomfortable symptoms, pause immediately and consult a professional. Safety is always the priority.
- **Switch:** If your sleep has stabilized but you've been stuck in a fat-loss plateau for over three weeks, it's time to make an adjustment. You can either transition from Starter A to Starter B, or take a short maintenance break before beginning a new cycle. This strategy prevents burnout and maintains metabolic responsiveness.
- **Sustain:** Once you have achieved your target body composition and optimal energy balance, shift into a maintenance phase. The goal here is to protect your results, not push harder. Continue resistance training, maintain steady protein intake, and treat high-quality sleep as your lifelong "forever stack".

Advanced Strategies for Stubborn Plateaus

If, after eight consistent weeks, your photos and waist measurements stop changing, but your mood, energy, and sleep are all stable, you can try these advanced, fine-tuning adjustments:

- **Step-Ladder Deficit:** Cycle between days of modest calorie deficit and maintenance days (e.g., three days at a 15% calorie deficit followed by one maintenance day). This technique helps prevent metabolic slowdown and keeps training intensity and thyroid function responsive.
- **Carb Cycling Around Lifts:** Increase your carbohydrate intake on training days, especially in the meals before and after lifting, and reduce them on rest days. This supports performance, stabilizes hormones, and sustains fat-burning momentum throughout the week.

- **Non-Exercise Activity Thermogenesis (NEAT) Pulse:** For 10–14 days, add a simple 30-minute walk after dinner each evening. This gentle increase in NEAT Pulse often restarts progress without requiring a change to your meal plan.
- **Deload Week:** If motivation drops or your joints feel achy, reduce your training intensity for 5–7 days, but ensure you maintain your protein intake and step count. This recovery-focused reset often leads to renewed strength gains and fat loss when normal training resumes.

REMEMBER

Plateaus are data, not a defeat. The smartest move is to adjust intelligently, rather than pushing harder.

Measurement Protocol (So Results Are Obvious)

Tracking your progress converts your effort into tangible evidence. Consistent measurement ensures that even small changes are visible, which keeps you motivated and allows for informed adjustments.

Frequency	Metrics to Track
Weekly	Waist measurement at the navel; Front, side, and back progress photos; Average morning weight (using a 3-day rolling average); Strength check on one key lifting exercise.
Daily	Sleep quality rating; Total step count; Protein intake in grams; Hunger and cravings on a 1–10 scale.
Every 4 Weeks	Notes on how clothing fits (belt hole, pants, or dress size); Overall mood summary; Average energy level.

Combining these daily, weekly, and monthly tracking methods provides an undeniable record of progress. This makes results visible even when the scale moves slowly, strengthening your confidence and consistency.

Frequently Asked Questions

Q: Can I fast while using these stacks?

A: Light time-restricted eating can be incorporated if you ensure you maintain adequate calories and protein. Avoid extreme fasting, which can compromise lean-mass preservation and sleep quality.

Q: What if I can't tolerate AOD-9604?

A: Focus on the night signaling with CJC-1295 + Ipamorelin and rely on the Meal Plan's strategic carbohydrate timing. Many people achieve excellent results without the morning cues once their recovery and sleep have stabilized.

Q: How long should a fat-loss cycle last?

A: Typical cycles run for 8–12 weeks. Follow this with at least a two-week break for maintenance before starting a new cycle to protect your energy and hormones.

Q: Do women respond differently?

A: Yes. Women often notice improvements in their sleep quality and waist measurements before any changes appear on the scale. Resistance training and high-protein intake are particularly vital for preserving lean mass in women.

Q: What if I'm traveling?

A: Prioritize your protein intake, consistent bedtime, and daily steps. If injections are impractical, pause your cycle and restart it when you return. Maintaining sleep patterns is the best defense against regression.

Fat-loss stacks are most effective when paired with flexibility, consistency, and smart habits. Adjustments are normal, and progress is driven by tracking, not striving for perfection.

Metabolic Myths to Retire

Dispelling common fat-loss beliefs that do more harm than good allows you to work smarter.

Myth	Reality
"No pain, no gain."	Your nervous system must feel safe to release fat. Calm, restorative sleep is a far better metabolic support than punishing, intense early-morning workouts.
"Cardio melts fat."	Cardio is helpful, but maintaining muscle is the key factor for a strong metabolic rate. Prioritize resistance training first, then add walks or Zone-2 activity.
"The scale is the truth."	Changes in body composition often become visible long before significant scale movement. Track clothing fit and waist measurements for a clearer picture of your progress.
"Cutting carbs is the only way."	Carbohydrates, when timed appropriately around workouts, protect performance, preserve lean mass, and support quality sleep while still enabling fat loss.

Second Mini Story: Elena's Midsection Breakthrough

Elena, a 52-year-old experienced runner, struggled with persistent belly fat despite regularly running half-marathons. She made strategic changes: she added two weekly resistance training sessions, slowed her longest runs to a Zone-2 pace, and began Starter Stack B. Tracking in her Journal confirmed the changes: her sleep improved within 10 days. By week 6, she had lost only four pounds but her waist had shrunk by two inches. Her body had visibly recomposed, not just lost weight. Elena's story demonstrates that a combination of smart stacking, consistent tracking, and strategic movement can create meaningful, visible changes without the need for extreme cardio or restrictive dieting.

Hormone Harmony Considerations for Men & Women 35+

Peptides are powerful tools, but they work within your overall hormonal context. For anyone experiencing early andropause or navigating perimenopause/postmenopause, the foundation is non-negotiable: prioritize quality sleep, commit to resistance training, and maintain a consistent, high protein intake. Peptides can assist with fat mobilization, collagen production, and GH rhythm, but they cannot compensate for a system that is severely under-nourished or sleep-deprived. Addressing basic health factors first will multiply the effectiveness of peptides. If you suspect underlying issues like thyroid problems or iron/vitamin deficiencies, work with a clinician.

Signals to Monitor:

- Hair thinning
- Depressed mood
- Low morning energy
- Cold intolerance
- Night sweats
- Lowered libido

These signals don't prevent peptide use, but they suggest that a slower, more stable approach is needed, with extra focus on recovery and supporting micronutrients (like iodine, selenium, B12, vitamin D, and zinc) as guided by lab work.

Diet Breaks Without Derailing Progress

A diet break is a planned maintenance period of 7–14 days that follows a typical 8–12 week fat-loss cycle. It's not a chance to overeat; it's a necessary signal to your nervous system that your body is safe and well-nourished.

During this pause, the following occurs:

- Appetite hormones are given a chance to recalibrate.
- Training performance often rebounds.
- Sleep quality tends to improve.

Guidelines for a Successful Break:

- Keep your protein intake high to safeguard lean mass.
- Maintain your daily step count and resistance training routine.
- Resume a gentle calorie deficit immediately after the break.

Many individuals find that these strategic breaks actually enhance long-term fat loss because the body exits its conservation mode and becomes more responsive to the next cycle.

Environment Setup Checklist: Make the Easy Choice the Right Choice

Setting up your environment to support your goals eliminates guesswork and promotes habit consistency. Small changes make the healthy option the most obvious and effortless one.

Key Setup Steps:

- **Protein Ready:** Keep pre-cooked options (like turkey meatballs, rotisserie chicken, or salmon) stocked for quick meals.
- **Visible Produce:** Place healthy options (like berries, baby carrots, cherry tomatoes, and cucumbers) at eye level for easy snacking.
- **Portion Nuts**: Pre-portion nuts into single-serving bags and store them out of immediate reach to prevent overconsumption.
- **Hydration Prep:** Fill a large water bottle every morning and set a goal to finish it before dinner.
- **Kitchen Curfew:** Use a timer to close the kitchen 3 hours before bed to protect your GH pulses.
- **Workout & Tracking Reminders:** Place your journal and pen on the nightstand, and your walking shoes near the door for easy access.

Design your physical space to reinforce your daily biological signals. When healthy habits are effortless, consistency improves, and your body receives clear messages for recovery, energy, and fat loss.

Example Week Schedule: Putting It Together

This sample week demonstrates how to strategically coordinate peptides, training, and nutrition to maximize their effect while prioritizing consistency and recovery.

Day	Routine
Monday	Resistance A + Meal Plan training day + Starter stack at night
Tuesday	40-minute walk + mobility work + AOD-9604 in the morning
Wednesday	Resistance B + optional light intervals + Starter stack at night
Thursday	45-minute walk after dinner + earlier cutoff for caffeine
Friday	Resistance A + higher-carb dinner timed post-training
Saturday	Long Zone-2 walk with family + meal prep for the week + lights out by 10:30 PM
Sunday	Off day + review Journal entries + plan the upcoming week + note a non-scale win

Understanding Resistance A and B Workouts

Your Resistance A and Resistance B workouts work together as a simple, powerful system to help you build lean muscle, support peptide signaling, and boost your metabolism without overtraining or burnout.

Resistance A: Foundation and Posterior Chain

Resistance A is your base-building workout. It targets the back side of your body, including your core, glutes, hamstrings, and back. These muscles drive posture, strength, and fat burning.

Goals of Resistance A:

- Stimulate growth hormone naturally through large compound lifts.
- Build lean, functional muscle for strength and joint support.
- Enhance insulin sensitivity and metabolic flexibility.

Resistance B: Upper Body and Anterior Chain

Resistance B complements your A workout by focusing on the front side of the body, such as the chest, shoulders, arms, and quads. These movements balance your posture and build visible tone and definition.

Goals of Resistance B:

- Strengthen upper-body pushing muscles including the chest, shoulders, and triceps.
- Improve core stability and symmetry through balanced muscle activation.
- Reinforce peptide-driven recovery and repair between sessions.

How They Work Together

Alternating Resistance A and B creates a **balanced, full-body program** that keeps your **hormonal and peptide signals aligned** with your workouts. You train all major muscle groups efficiently, activate muscle growth, improve recovery, and support steady fat loss without overloading your system.

What Success Feels Like

Success goes far beyond the number on the scale. You will begin to notice a sense of cooperation from your body, calmer evenings, and less pressure surrounding food. Your joints will feel more comfortable, your clothes will fit better, and training sessions will be more productive. The mirror will start to reflect firmer, healthier lines where they matter most. This feeling of partnering with your own physiology is the ultimate reward of peptide-supported fat loss.

With improved recovery and fat loss underway, the next critical step is protecting and rebuilding lean muscle, which is the "currency of longevity". The next chapter will cover how to:

- Stack signals effectively for strength gains.
- Leverage sleep to enhance performance.
- Follow a four-week rebuild plan that secures your newly optimized metabolism.

While visible results are important, the most lasting transformation comes from the confidence, energy, and harmony you establish with your body.

CHAPTER 4

LEAN MUSCLE POWER: REBUILD STRENGTH, PROTECT METABOLISM, AND AGE STRONG

When it comes to lasting transformation, muscle is your secret weapon. It's not just about looking toned, it's about feeling strong, balanced, and alive. Fat loss may start the process, but muscle keeps the fire burning. As we age, stress, poor recovery, and restrictive habits chip away at lean mass, slowing down metabolism and making it harder to stay fit. The good news? You can rebuild that foundation.

- Fat loss sparks change, but muscle sustains it.
- Muscle fuels metabolism, hormones, and joint protection.
- After 35, lean mass naturally declines by about 1 percent each year.
- Stress, under-eating, and excessive cardio speed up muscle loss.
- Peptides help reactivate recovery and muscle growth pathways.

By supporting your body's natural repair signals, you can rebuild strength, improve energy, and move with confidence. Peptides don't replace the work; they make the work work better.

Why Muscle Is Your Real Youth Hormone

Muscle isn't just about strength or looks; it's the body's built-in youth signal. Every time you move, lift, or carry, you're telling your biology: "Stay functional, stay alive." Muscle tissue drives your metabolism, balances blood sugar, and stabilizes hormones. The more you preserve and challenge it, the longer your body keeps running like it's years younger. Building or maintaining muscle is not vanity; it's your most powerful anti-aging investment.

Benefit	Mechanism	Felt Result
Higher metabolic rate	Increases resting energy expenditure	Easier weight maintenance
Better glucose control	Improves insulin sensitivity	Fewer energy crashes
Stronger bones	Raises mechanical loading	Lower fracture risk
Balanced mood	Releases myokines and endorphins	Less anxiety and depression
Longevity signaling	Stimulates AMPK (energy sensor) and mTOR rhythm (growth switch)	Slower biological aging

Muscle acts like your body's renewable youth hormone, fueling metabolism, protecting mood, and keeping your internal clock running younger. Every rep is a signal to keep thriving.

Why Traditional Workouts Stop Working

When it comes to midlife fitness, effort isn't the issue; strategy is. Many people still follow workout routines built on outdated ideas: endless cardio, familiar machines, and weights that never change. These routines can initially feel productive, but quickly lose their effectiveness. The real challenge isn't consistency; it's communication. Your body listens to signals, not habits. Once those signals become stale, progress stalls, and fatigue takes over, replacing growth.

Here's what's really happening:

- Your body adapts fast. Repeating the same workouts sends no new message to grow or rebuild.

- Without progressive overload, there's no reason for your muscles to get stronger or denser.
- Lack of proper recovery time keeps your repair systems constantly behind schedule.
- Missing nutrients mean even good workouts don't translate into visible change.
- Overdoing cardio can blunt muscle-building signals and slow metabolism over time.

Where peptides come in:
Peptides act like a refresh button for your system. They help your cells become more responsive, make recovery more efficient, deepen your sleep, and strengthen your body's protein-building process.
Real progress at midlife is not about pushing harder; it's about restoring communication between effort and adaptation.

Meet the Rebuild Stack (Your Muscle Signal Trio)

Think of this stack as a support team for your workouts. Each peptide plays a distinct role in helping your body recover, rebuild, and maintain lean mass. Together, they strengthen the signals that drive growth, mobility, and long-term joint health, especially when paired with consistent resistance training and proper nutrition.

1) CJC-1295 + Ipamorelin (Bedtime Recovery Duo)
- Stimulates nightly growth hormone pulses that fuel muscle repair and fat metabolism.
- Eases joint stress from heavy lifting and daily movement.
- Expect better sleep, faster recovery, and more steady morning energy within 2–3 weeks.

2) BPC-157 (Daytime Support & Tissue Repair)
- Speeds healing in tendons, joints, and connective tissues, great for knees, shoulders, and elbows.
- Works gently throughout the body and is suitable for extended use.
- Ideal for athletes or anyone recovering from training-related strain.

3) TB-500 (Circulation & Mobility Enhancer)

- Encourages the formation of new blood vessels, thereby improving nutrient delivery to muscle fibers.
- Supports flexibility, tissue repair, and overall mobility when combined with stretching and hydration.

The Rebuild Stack doesn't replace training; it amplifies your body's ability to adapt, recover, and stay strong for the long game.

Training Blueprint for Muscle Gain After 35

Your body still has incredible potential to build muscle; it just needs smarter signals. After the age of 35, recovery, hormones, and metabolism respond differently. This blueprint aligns the training structure, tempo, and recovery with how your physiology now functions most effectively. The goal isn't to train harder but to train intelligently, with consistency and precision.

Resistance Training (3–4×/week)

- Two full-body sessions plus two focused days (upper/lower split).
- Prioritize compound lifts: squat, hinge, push, pull, carry.
- Maintain high intensity, but prioritize form and control.

Progressive Overload

- Add small increases in weight, reps, or time under tension each week.
- Tiny adjustments can lead to significant body recomposition over 90 days.

Tempo & Control

- Use a 2-second lower, 1-second pause, and 1-second lift.
- Focus on tension and muscle connection over speed or ego lifting.

Rest & Recovery

- Allow at least 48 hours between intense sessions.
- Combine peptides, deep sleep, and optimal nutrient timing for accelerated recovery.

Walk Daily

- Gentle movement boosts circulation, recovery, and fat metabolism without overtaxing your system.

Consistency and controlled effort build momentum. Every rep is a message to your body: grow stronger, stay younger, keep moving.

Nutrition: Fuel for Growth

You can't rebuild muscle on fumes. Food is the raw material your body uses to recover, grow, and stabilize hormones. The goal here isn't to "bulk up" but to re-compose, building lean muscle, lowering fat, and keeping your body weight stable or slightly higher. With the proper fuel and timing, your peptides, training, and recovery signals all align for visible transformation.

Macros That Work

- **Protein:** 1 gram per pound of lean mass (or 30–40 g per meal). This is your repair foundation. Every muscle fiber depends on it.
- **Carbs:** Incorporate them into your workouts to replenish glycogen and support better sleep through serotonin balance.
- **Fats:** Keep 30–35% of calories from quality fats to maintain hormone function and joint health.

Sample Day (30-Day Meal Plan Preview – Muscle Phase)

- **Breakfast:** Protein pancakes topped with berries and a drizzle of Greek yogurt.
- **Lunch:** Grilled salmon bowl with rice, avocado, and spinach.
- **Snack:** Beef jerky with an apple.
- **Dinner:** Chicken stir-fry with jasmine rice and mixed vegetables.
- **Evening:** Cottage cheese with almond butter, steady protein to support nighttime GH pulses.

TIP

Check your Meal Plan PDF for personalized macros, grocery lists, and weekly protein rotation ideas to make adherence effortless.

Sleep: Your Anabolic Window

Sleep isn't passive recovery, it's the most powerful anabolic state your body enters each day. During deep sleep, growth hormone and IGF-1 surge, sending the message to repair, rebuild, and renew. This is when peptides like CJC-1295 + Ipamorelin do their best work, naturally enhancing those hormonal pulses to facilitate faster tissue repair, improved fat metabolism, and stronger muscle synthesis.

Aim for 7½ to 9 hours of quality sleep in a dark, cool, quiet room. Temperature and light both affect how deeply you cycle through REM and slow-wave stages. To prepare your body for rest, cut off screens at least an hour before bed. Blue light suppresses melatonin, so replace scrolling with light stretching, journaling, or reading.

If stress or racing thoughts make it hard to wind down, consider adding a short breathing practice (four-count inhale, six-count exhale) to lower cortisol before lights out.

Consistent, deep sleep multiplies the effect of every peptide and every rep you perform in training. It's not an optional recovery tool; it's the amplifier of all progress. Protecting your sleep routine is the simplest, most underrated performance enhancer you'll ever use.

Men vs Women: How Responses Differ

Peptides speak the same cellular language in everybody, but men and women often experience the effects differently. These differences aren't about fairness; they stem from hormonal environment, receptor density, and enzyme activity. Understanding these distinctions helps you set realistic expectations and optimize protocols for your physiology.

Aspect	Men	Women
Growth Hormone Pulses	Larger amplitude pulses	More frequent, smaller pulses
Estrogen Interaction	Enhances collagen & joint repair	Supports fat distribution changes
Recovery window	Slightly shorter	Benefits more from sleep and collagen support
Visual trend	Muscle definition first	Firmness & skin glow first

Regardless of gender, strength gains and body recomposition are achievable when protein intake, sleep, and recovery practices are consistently applied. The rhythm of response may differ, but the end result, improved performance, metabolism, and physique, is equally impressive.

The Journal Connection

Tracking progress is more than accountability. Your 30-Day Journal captures the data that predicts muscle gain and recovery efficiency. Recording consistently allows you to identify patterns, adjust your strategies, and stay motivated when results seem slow.

Key Metrics to Track:

- **Sleep:** Hours and quality each night.
- **Protein:** Total grams and meal timing.
- **Training:** Sessions completed, weights used, and progression in lifts.
- **Recovery Score:** Morning energy rated 1–10.

By the third week, patterns emerge. Higher protein intake aligns with faster recovery. Better sleep leads to stronger lifts. Small daily data points compound into actionable insights, guiding your next move in training and nutrition.

Mini Case Story: "The Comeback Year"

Tony, 49, had sidelined himself for months after a rotator-cuff injury. He began a rehabilitation plan that included **BPC-157** and light band exercises. By week six, he added **CJC + Ipamorelin** at night. Sleep improved to eight hours, and pain decreased by roughly 60 percent. By week twelve, he was pressing weights again with better form than before.

Tony's reflection captures the lesson: "I didn't get stronger by pushing harder; I got stronger by recovering better."

This story highlights how targeted peptides combined with smart recovery and progressive training can restore strength safely, even after setbacks, without relying on brute force.

Recovery Rituals That Multiply Growth

Muscle growth doesn't happen in the gym, it happens in recovery. Your body needs consistent signals, nutrients, and circulation to repair tissue, reduce inflammation, and prepare for the next training session. Combining intentional recovery habits with peptides amplifies results and protects long-term performance.

Key Recovery Habits:

- **Hydration:** Drink water early in the day; replenish electrolytes after training.
- **Temperature Therapy:** Use contrast showers or cold rinses after heavy sessions to reduce inflammation.
- **Evening Wind-Down:** Stretch and practice deep breathing for five minutes before bed to lower cortisol and support GH pulses.
- **Active Rest:** Light walks, mobility drills, or gentle movement on rest days help maintain strong circulation without overstressing muscles.
- **Peptide Pairing:** Support your recovery with BPC-157 and TB-500 to enhance tissue repair and nutrient delivery.

Recovery isn't passive; it's an active process that multiplies your training and peptide signals. A structured 24-hour repair loop ensures that your body rebuilds stronger, faster, and more efficiently, turning effort into lasting growth.

Hormone Synergy and Peptide Support

Peptides are powerful tools for boosting growth hormone rhythms, promoting recovery, and facilitating cellular repair, but they are not a magic solution. Think of them as amplifiers; they enhance the body's natural signals, but the quality of those signals depends on your own hormonal environment. For lean muscle growth, fat metabolism, stable mood, and consistent energy, sex hormones like testosterone, estrogen, and progesterone must be in balance. Growth hormones and peptides lay the groundwork, but your sex hormones determine how well that foundation translates into visible results.

Why Hormones Still Matter:

- **Men:** Low testosterone can limit peptide-driven muscle gain, slow recovery, and contribute to fatigue, low motivation, and stubborn belly fat.
- **Women:** Imbalances in estrogen or progesterone can impair sleep, mood, and fat loss. Excess estrogen may cause water retention and sluggish progress.
- **Peptide Limitation:** Peptides enhance the system they enter; they do not override hormonal imbalances.

Signs of Hormonal Imbalance:

- Low libido or reduced morning energy
- Flat mood or emotional blunting
- Poor post-workout recovery
- Sleep disturbances or night sweats
- Unexplained weight gain or loss of muscle tone

Steps to Restore Synergy:

- Prioritize quality sleep (7–9 hours), protein-rich meals, and resistance training to stabilize hormone rhythms.

- Optimize key micronutrients, including zinc, magnesium, vitamin D, and omega-3 fatty acids, which support hormone production and peptide signaling.
- Collaborate with a knowledgeable clinician for bioidentical or microdose hormone support guided by lab results.
- Track improvements in energy, sleep, mood, and body composition as feedback loops to inform future decisions.

Peptides are most effective when paired with a healthy, balanced hormonal system. When hormones, lifestyle, and peptides work together, your body functions like a symphony instead of a solo. Proper alignment multiplies results safely and sustainably.

This content is for educational purposes only. *Consult a qualified healthcare professional before starting any peptide or hormone regimen.*

How to Periodize Your Muscle Plan

Optimizing muscle growth isn't just about lifting heavier each week. It's about aligning your training intensity with recovery, nutrition, and peptide signaling. Periodization helps you progressively challenge your muscles while preventing burnout and maximizing results. Structuring your cycles ensures your peptides enhance the right processes at the right time, from skill acquisition to peak performance and recovery.

Phase Overview:

- **Reset (Weeks 1–2):** Focus on technique, mobility, and foundational movement patterns. Use CJC-1295 + Ipamorelin only to support nightly growth hormone pulses and sleep-driven recovery.
- **Build (Weeks 3–6):** Increase load and progressive overload. Add BPC-157 to accelerate tissue repair and maintain tendon and joint health under growing stress.
- **Peak (Weeks 7–10):** Emphasize intensity and training volume. Optionally include TB-500 to enhance circulation, nutrient delivery, and flexibility for harder sessions.

- **Deload (Weeks 11–12):** Prioritize recovery, sleep, and nervous system reset. Pause most peptides except BPC-157 if ongoing tissue support is needed.

A deload is a scheduled recovery phase where you reduce training stress to let your body fully repair. It helps reset your nervous system, lower inflammation, and improve long-term results.

Following this periodized approach allows your training, nutrition, and peptides to work in harmony. Each phase prepares your body for the next, making growth sustainable, minimizing injury risk, and ensuring the results you build are preserved long-term. Aligning cycles with a specific plan simplifies tracking and keeps your body operating efficiently.

Advanced Muscle & Recomposition Stack (Experienced Users Only)

For those who have completed foundational cycles and understand peptide timing, this stack maximizes lean-muscle gain, recovery, and body recomposition. It leverages complementary peptides to amplify natural growth signals, accelerate tissue repair, and enhance circulation. Pairing these signals with proper nutrition, resistance training, and recovery routines ensures safety and measurable results.

Stack Components:

- **CJC-1295 + Ipamorelin (Bedtime):** Boosts nighttime GH pulses, improving protein synthesis, fat mobilization, and joint recovery.
- **BPC-157 (Morning):** Supports soft-tissue repair, reduces micro-inflammation, and enhances tendon and ligament resilience.
- **TB-500 (Every Other Week):** Promotes angiogenesis, improves nutrient delivery to muscles, and enhances mobility.

Cycle:

- **Duration:** 12 weeks active → 2 weeks off to allow receptor sensitivity reset and support long-term response.

Support Strategies:

- Follow a high-protein Meal Plan to sustain repair and lean mass gains.

- Track workouts, recovery, and sleep using the Journal to monitor subtle trends and patterns.

Expected Results:

- Noticeable muscle firmness and shape improvements by week 6.
- Enhanced recovery between sessions.
- Reduced joint or tissue discomfort during higher-volume training blocks.

NOTE

This is intended for experienced users familiar with peptide timing, dosing, and training alignment. Always consult a qualified clinician before use.

Mindset Shift: Train for Functional Strength

Building strength after 35 is about more than appearance, it's about capability. Each lift, carry, or hike reinforces your body's ability to move, recover, and remain independent. Functional strength protects joints, improves posture, supports metabolic health, and makes daily life easier. Training with this mindset shifts focus from aesthetics to resilience, longevity, and measurable performance.

Journal Prompts / Reflection:

- What movement or lift today felt easier than last week? Track progress beyond the scale.
- How did last night's sleep influence today's workout performance and recovery?
- Which exercise made me feel capable, strong, and energized?

Key Mindset Points:

- Strength is cumulative: small, consistent improvements compound over weeks and months.
- Every training session is a vote for your future mobility and independence.
- Capability beats perfection; form, recovery, and consistency matter more than ego or weight lifted.

Adopting this perspective helps maintain high motivation, reduces burnout, and reinforces a positive feedback loop: better sleep, stronger lifts, faster recovery, and increased confidence in daily life. Training becomes a practice in longevity, not just muscle.

Mini Story: "Lydia's Strong Again Moment"

Lydia, 57, had avoided weights for years due to chronic back pain. Her coach introduced gentle banded hinges paired with nightly CJC + Ipamorelin for recovery. Within just one month, she slept through the night without painkillers. By week 8, she was confidently deadlifting 65 pounds and smiling through every rep. In her Journal, she wrote: "For the first time, my body feels capable again."

Checklist, Your First Four Weeks of Rebuild

- Follow Meal Plan Weeks 5–8 (muscle phase)
- Use Bedtime Stack nightly
- Lift 3–4×/week
- Walk daily
- Sleep 7–9 hours
- Record metrics in the Journal every night

Consistency is more important than perfection. Small, daily efforts compound into real functional strength, better sleep, and higher energy. Tracking progress with a Journal keeps motivation high and makes gains visible beyond the scale.

With strength restored and recovery improving, it's time to protect joints and mobility for the long term. Chapter 5 will guide you through Pain Repair Power, showing you how to utilize BPC-157, TB-500, and supportive nutrition to keep your movements pain-free while extending your active, capable years.

CHAPTER 5

JOINT & PAIN REPAIR POWER: HEAL, MOVE BETTER, AND STAY ACTIVE FOR LIFE

When joints ache or tendons burn, everything shrinks, your workouts, confidence, and even mood. After 35, collagen turnover slows, recovery stretches out, and small injuries that once healed overnight can linger for weeks.

Protecting and repairing connective tissue isn't optional, it's foundational to staying active and pain-free. By supporting tendon, ligament, and joint health, you preserve mobility, maintain workout consistency, and prevent minor aches from derailing your progress. This chapter lays out strategies to reverse age-related tissue decline, emphasizing peptides, nutrition, and targeted movement so your body recovers faster and moves easier.

Follow the tools and protocols here to rebuild resilience. With consistent care, you can lift, walk, and live without fear of setbacks, turning every session into a confidence-building win and extending your active years.

Why Joints Need Special Attention After 35

Cartilage has almost no direct blood supply, so its repair relies on good circulation, proper hydration, and consistent movement. Years of repetitive stress from sitting, running, or lifting with poor form can create tiny tears that outpace the body's repair capacity. Hormonal changes that thin collagen fibers make knees, shoulders, and lower backs more prone to discomfort.

Supporting joint health isn't just about avoiding pain, it's about restoring the body's natural repair signals. Peptides act as precise messengers, telling cells when and where to rebuild, while protein, collagen, and essential minerals provide the raw materials needed for tissue recovery. Combining these with consistent, targeted movement ensures that repair keeps pace with daily wear and tear.

Use the strategies in this chapter to reinforce cartilage, tendons, and ligaments. When you supply the right signals and substrates, you can maintain mobility, protect your workouts, and prevent small aches from turning into chronic issues. Healthy joints are the foundation for freedom of movement well into your later years.

The Repair Signal Team

Supporting joint, tendon, and ligament health requires precise signals and consistent substrates. These peptides work synergistically to speed repair, reduce inflammation, and improve mobility.

1) BPC-157 : The Tissue Healer

- Derived from a gastric protein that protects the gut and soft tissues.
- Promotes fibroblast growth and angiogenesis for better nutrient delivery.
- Reduces inflammation and pain sensitivity in tendons and ligaments.
- Timing: 1–2 times daily for 8–12 weeks depending on injury severity.
- Expected: Noticeable improvement in mobility within 7–10 days.

2) TB-500: The Mobility Messenger

- Mimics thymosin beta-4 to enhance cell migration and tissue remodeling.
- Supports circulation and reduces fibrosis (scar tissue buildup).
- Timing: Every other week micro dose for 8 weeks.
- Expected: Looser, smoother movement by week 3.

3) GH-Support (CJC + Ipamorelin)

- Amplifies nightly growth hormone pulses to stimulate collagen synthesis and recovery.
- Works best combined with BPC-157 or TB-500 for structural repair acceleration.

These three signals form a coordinated repair team. BPC-157 targets tissue healing, TB-500 enhances mobility, and GH-support ensures collagen production and recovery are optimized. Together, they help your joints and connective tissues recover faster, stay flexible, and support long-term movement freedom.

Integrate these peptides with protein-rich meals, collagen sources, hydration, and gentle movement. This combination maximizes repair, prevents setbacks, and keeps your body resilient to the demands of daily life and training.

Nutrition for Joint Rebuild

Peptides provide the instructions, but raw materials build the tissue. Collagen, amino acids, vitamins, minerals, and healthy fats are essential for repairing tendons, ligaments, and cartilage. Without proper nutrition, even the best signaling can't produce resilient joints.

Joint Rebuild Essentials

- **Protein:** 1 g per pound of lean mass minimum. Include 10–15 g collagen powder daily in coffee, shakes, or snacks.
- **Vitamin C:** Critical for collagen cross-linking. Add citrus, bell peppers, or kiwi to meals.
- **Omega-3s:** 2 g EPA + DHA daily to reduce inflammation and joint discomfort.
- **Hydration:** Aim for half your body weight in ounces of water daily, plus electrolytes if sweating.
- **Anti-Inflammatory Spices:** Turmeric with black pepper, ginger, and garlic incorporated into meals.

Sample Day (Joint Phase)

- **Breakfast:** Collagen latte + egg scramble with spinach and avocado.
- **Lunch:** Salmon wrap with mixed greens and olive-oil dressing.
- **Snack:** Greek yogurt + berries + chia seeds.
- **Dinner:** Roasted chicken thighs with quinoa and broccoli.
- **Evening:** Chamomile tea + collagen peptide scoop.

Think of your nutrition as construction materials for your connective tissue. Protein and collagen provide building blocks, vitamin C cements the structure, and omega-3s and anti-inflammatory spices reduce repair roadblocks.

Pair this nutrition strategy with your peptide protocol and recovery rituals. Together, they create a strong, flexible foundation, helping joints tolerate training, reduce pain, and stay resilient for years to come.

Mobility & Movement Plan

Healing isn't just about rest, it's about smart, controlled movement. Gentle, pain-free motion stimulates blood flow, delivers nutrients to connective tissue, and prevents stiffness. Staying too still slows repair and reduces the effectiveness of peptides and nutrition.

POWER ROUTINE: Daily Joint Flow (10 Minutes)

This 10-minute sequence keeps joints mobile, connective tissue nourished, and recovery optimized. Pair with your peptide support and protein-rich meals for maximal tissue repair.

Flow:

- **Cat-Cow (×10):** Slowly arch and round your spine to loosen the back, activate the core, and stimulate spinal circulation.
- **Shoulder Circles (×20):** Roll shoulders forward and backward to release tension and improve upper-body posture.
- **Hip 90/90 Rotations (×10 each side):** Sit with knees at right angles, rotate gently side to side to open hips and glutes.

- **Ankle Alphabets (A–Z):** "Write" the alphabet with your toes to strengthen ankles, enhance stability, and promote blood flow.
- **Standing Reach & Twist (×10):** Reach overhead, twist gently left and right while breathing deeply, re-aligns the spine and boosts circulation.

Finisher:

- Spend 3 minutes in deep nasal breathing to lower cortisol, a key barrier to tissue repair and joint recovery.

When to Use:

- Daily, either in the morning, pre-workout, or on recovery days.
- Consistency helps your peptides, nutrition, and training synergize, accelerating joint resilience and overall mobility.

This routine is simple but powerful; it primes your body for activity, reduces stiffness, and supports long-term joint health.

Pain is Information, Not Punishment

It's your body's way of saying, *"Pay attention here."* By pairing mindful movement with targeted peptide support, you help your system recognize the difference between injury and stiffness, between protection and limitation. The goal isn't to silence pain, it's to translate it. When you understand pain as a signal instead of a sentence, you respond with care, not fear, and that's where true healing begins.

Power Prompt for Your Journal:

- Which movement felt smoother or easier today compared to last week?
- What small habit, stretch, or nutrition tweak contributed to that improvement?

Viewing pain as a signal allows you to stay active safely, prioritize recovery, and make informed adjustments. Over time, your joints become more resilient, connective tissue stronger, and your confidence in movement grows.

The Repair Timeline

Healing takes consistency, not speed. With peptide support, proper nutrition, and targeted movement, your joints and connective tissue gradually regain strength and flexibility. Tracking progress weekly helps you see small wins that add up to full recovery without rushing or risking setbacks.

Week	What to Expect	Action Step
1	Reduced morning stiffness	Stay hydrated, track sleep hours
2	Soreness decreases, range improves	Add 10-minute mobility flow each morning
3–4	Noticeable pain reduction	Begin light strength sessions
5–6	Strength returns	Maintain peptide protocol, increase load gradually
7–8	Full movement confidence	Re-introduce sport or higher-intensity activity

Use this timeline as a guide, not a race. Consistent hydration, mobility, and peptide cycles compound to accelerate repair. Celebrate each milestone and only progress intensity when your body signals readiness.

Mini Story: "Running Without Fear"

Maya, 44, a teacher and weekend runner, developed knee pain that forced her to stop training. Her clinician introduced BPC-157 alongside collagen supplementation and twice-weekly strength sessions. Within three weeks, she was jogging 15 minutes pain-free. By week 8, she completed a 5K without discomfort. In her journal, she reflected: "The freedom to run again is worth every injection."
This story highlights how targeted peptide support, combined with proper nutrition and strength training, can restore mobility and confidence safely.

POWER RECOVERY, Advanced Strategies for Chronic Pain

Even with consistent peptide use, chronic pain can linger. This does not mean your protocol failed, it means your body is still working through deeper layers of inflammation, nutrient gaps, or stress. Peptides accelerate repair, but they need the right environment to complete the job. Use this 5-step synergy system to restore healing momentum.

1. Calm Gut Inflammation (The Hidden Pain Trigger)

A sluggish or inflamed gut keeps your immune system "on alert," draining recovery hormones and stalling collagen repair.

Why it matters: The gut is your recovery command center, if it's inflamed, peptides can't work optimally.

What to do:

- Simplify meals for 14–21 days, remove gluten, alcohol, seed oils, and processed sugars.
- Add bone broth, leafy greens, omega-3s, and probiotics.
- Support peptides like BPC-157 and TB-500 with gut-healing nutrients (zinc carnosine, glutamine, ginger, turmeric).
- **Power Pair:** BPC-157 + anti-inflammatory nutrition = accelerated tendon and gut lining repair.

2. Reset Cortisol and Stress Hormones (The GH Blocker)

Chronic stress keeps cortisol high, blunting GH pulses and dulling peptide signaling.

Why it matters: Without rest, the body cannot rebuild; it just survives.

What to do:

- Establish a nightly shutdown ritual (no screens, warm shower, magnesium glycinate, deep breathing).
- Consider Epitalon or DSIP to help restore circadian rhythm and deep sleep.
- Use gentle Zone-2 cardio or short post-meal walks to lower cortisol naturally.

Power Pair: CJC-1295 + Ipamorelin + consistent sleep = deeper recovery and reduced inflammation.

3. The Repair Materials (What Builders Need to Work)

Peptides are builders and they need the right materials to work.

Why it matters: Without amino acids, minerals, and vitamins, collagen synthesis and GH pathways slow.

What to do:

- Check labs for vitamin D, zinc, magnesium, and ferritin.
- Eat at least 1 g of protein per pound of goal body weight.
- Add collagen peptides, vitamin C, and copper to support tissue regeneration.

Power Pair: GHK-Cu + collagen-rich nutrition = stronger tendons, smoother skin, faster healing.

4. Correct Load Errors (The Overtraining Trap)

Pushing too hard too soon can reactivate inflammation and slow peptide progress.

Why it matters: Peptides speed recovery, but cannot prevent damage from overload.

What to do:

- Following progressive loading increases intensity or volume by ≤10% per week.
- Track soreness, sleep, and mood; if recovery lags, deload for 3–5 days.
- Use BPC-157 or TB-500 through gradual reloading phases to protect tissue integrity.

Power Pair: BPC-157 + strategic rest = long-term tendon and joint resilience.

5. Partner with a Qualified Clinician (The Optimization Step)

If pain persists beyond 8–10 weeks, deeper layers such as hormones, alignment, or autoimmune inflammation may be involved.

Why it matters: Personalized insight unlocks results you can't see from the outside.

What to do:

- Ask for a comprehensive panel: hormones, thyroid, CRP, insulin, micronutrients.
- Seek a clinician familiar with peptide therapy and functional medicine.

Power Pair: Medical oversight + customized stack cycle = long-term repair and functional freedom.

THE COMPLETE PAIN RELIEF SYNERGY STACK

Goal	Peptides	Lifestyle Support	Duration
Tendon / Ligament Repair	BPC-157 (250–500 mcg daily), TB-500 (2–5 mg weekly)	Gentle resistance training + high-protein meals	8–12 weeks
Inflammation & Recovery	GHK-Cu (supports skin & joint regeneration), Epitalon (cell renewal)	7–9 hours of quality sleep, reduce stressors	6–8 weeks
Chronic Overuse or Muscle Pain	CJC-1295 + Ipamorelin	3× weekly resistance sessions + rest days	8–12 weeks
Sleep / Nerve Pain	DSIP or Epitalon	Nighttime wind-down routine	6–8 weeks

Key Notes:

- Each stack is designed to target a specific pain or recovery pathway.
- Peptides work best when paired with the appropriate lifestyle support, including sleep, nutrition, and movement.
- Duration reflects typical cycles; reassess progress and recovery at the end of each period.

Disclaimer: *This information is for educational purposes only. It is not a substitute for medical advice. Always consult a qualified healthcare professional before starting any peptide, supplement, or therapy protocol.*

Stack Example, Repair & Recover Stack A

- **Peptides:** BPC-157 (daily), TB-500 (every other week)
- **Cycle:** 8–12 weeks, followed by a 2-week break
- **Pair With:** Joint-focused Meal Plan + Daily Mobility Protocol

Tips:

- Hydrate well before injections
- Perform daily stretching and mobility exercises
- Track pain and movement improvements in your Journal (1–10 scale)

This stack supports tendon, ligament, and soft tissue repair while improving joint mobility. Combining peptide signaling with proper nutrition, hydration, and movement maximizes recovery outcomes.

Mindset Shift, From Pain Avoidance to Movement Confidence

Healing isn't about never feeling discomfort. It's about relearning trust in your body. Every time you bend, twist, or lift without hesitation, you reinforce that your joints, muscles, and connective tissues are capable. This trust fuels motivation, consistency, and long-term progress. The goal of Joint & Pain Repair Power isn't just symptom relief, it's restoring confidence in movement so you can reclaim freedom in everyday life.

Focus on small wins, pain-free steps, smoother rotations, or reduced stiffness. Each success is a signal that your recovery plan, peptides, and lifestyle strategies are working together.

True movement confidence is the marker of progress. When you pair structural repair with consistent habits and mindful tracking, you don't just reduce pain, you gain the freedom to move, play, and live without limitations.

Checklist, Your 8-Week Joint Reset

Follow this routine consistently to maximize joint repair and recovery:

- Take BPC-157 daily as directed
- Administer TB-500 every other week
- Complete 10-minute Mobility Flow each day
- Meet protein and collagen targets
- Log hydration and omega-3 intake
- Sleep at least 7 hours per night
- Track weekly pain score in your Journal

Completing eight consistent weeks builds more than joint strength; it quiets the background aches that limit movement and confidence. Small daily actions compound into noticeable freedom, reduced soreness, and smoother mobility.

Once joints feel stable and mobility returns, you're ready to shift focus from recovery to rejuvenation. The next step, Skin & Collagen Renewal Power, leverages the same peptide and lifestyle principles to restore visible vitality in skin, hair, and connective tissue.

CHAPTER 6

SKIN, HAIR & BEAUTY FROM THE INSIDE OUT: COLLAGEN RENEWAL FOR VISIBLE VITALITY

After 35, it's common to notice fine lines, dull tone, slower hair growth, or skin that doesn't bounce back. You didn't suddenly "age", your collagen economy just tightened its budget.

This chapter shows how to restore that economy by upgrading your body's messages to build, protect, and remodel the tissues that define visible vitality: your skin, hair, nails, and the connective matrix beneath them.

This isn't a "cosmetic quick fix" chapter. It's a systems approach:

- **Signal:** Activate repair with targeted peptides
- **Support:** Nourish from within through nutrition and topical care
- **Stack:** Combine protocols strategically for synergy
- **Sustain:** Keep results through daily habits

When those four align, your reflection naturally follows.

POWER BEAUTY BOX: Why Skin Changes After 35 (and What You Can Do About It)

Your skin isn't just a surface, it's a living, responsive organ that renews itself every day.

Until your mid-30s, your skin's repair crew, **fibroblasts,** work tirelessly to produce collagen, elastin, and moisture-binding molecules that keep your complexion firm, smooth, and luminous.
But time, stress, UV exposure, disrupted sleep, and hormonal shifts

slow those builders down. Collagen begins breaking down faster than it's replaced. The scaffolding beneath your skin weakens, and the visible signs follow: fine lines, loss of tone, uneven texture.

The answer isn't to attack the surface harder, it's to **re-energize your builders** and feed them from the inside out. That's where **peptides shine,** by reigniting your skin's own renewal system.

THE SCIENCE: Why Collagen Declines

Cause	What Happens	Visible Effect
UV + Blue-Light Exposure	Damages DNA and weakens collagen fibers	Fine lines, rough texture
Poor Sleep / High Cortisol	Reduces growth hormone and fibroblast activity	Dull, tired complexion
Chronic Inflammation / Sugar	Cross-links collagen (glycation)	Loss of firmness, uneven tone
Hormonal Shifts (↓ Estrogen / GH)	Slows fibroblast signaling	Thinner, sagging skin
Nutrient Gaps (Vit C, Zinc, Copper)	Weak collagen synthesis	Slower healing, dull tone

Inside your skin, fibroblasts are your construction crews. They produce:

- Collagen for strength
- Elastin for flexibility
- Glycosaminoglycans (like hyaluronic acid) for bounce and moisture

Over time, their communication weakens, fewer "make more collagen" signals are sent, and renewal gradually slows. The goal of the next section is to restart those messages and retrain your skin to rebuild from within.

THE SOLUTION: Peptide Power Stack for Skin Renewal

Peptides are microscopic messengers that reawaken fibroblasts and restore the biological "conversation" of youth.

They don't force your skin to change, they remind it how to rebuild, repair, and renew naturally.

Peptide	Core Action	When to Use
GHK-Cu	Signals collagen + elastin rebuild, improves blood flow, brightens tone	AM/PM topical or injection, 5× weekly
Epitalon	Resets sleep cycles for deeper nighttime repair	PM before bed, 4–6-week cycles
Thymosin Beta-4 (TB-4)	Speeds micro-healing, boosts circulation, reduces redness	Ideal after skin stress or recovery weeks
CJC-1295 + Ipamorelin	Restores GH pulses, accelerates full-body tissue renewal	3–5× weekly (bedtime)

PRO TIP

Combine GHK-Cu (topical) with CJC-1295 + Ipamorelin (systemic) for the most complete inside–out skin regeneration synergy.

LIFESTYLE BOOSTERS: Feed the Builders

Habit	Benefit
Hydrate deeply: ½ body weight (oz/day)	Keeps skin matrix supple, oxygenated, and elastic
7–9 hours of sleep nightly	Collagen rebuild and growth hormone peak during deep sleep
1 g protein per pound of goal weight	Supplies amino acids that fuel fibroblast repair activity
Vitamin C + Zinc + Copper	Essential for collagen cross-linking and antioxidant protection
SPF + Antioxidants (Vitamin C serum, green tea, resveratrol)	Shields skin from oxidative damage and prevents new collagen loss

REMEMBER

Peptides amplify what's already healthy.

The stronger your foundation of nutrition, hydration, and rest, the greater your visible transformation.

VISIBLE RESULTS TIMELINE

Timeframe	What You'll Notice
Weeks 2–4	Skin feels smoother and more hydrated; a gentle, healthy glow returns
Weeks 4–8	Fine lines soften, firmness improves, and tone brightens noticeably
Weeks 8–12	Jawline and cheeks appear subtly lifted; deeper elasticity restored
Beyond 12 Weeks	Continuous collagen remodeling, visible youthful density and long-lasting luminosity

NOTE

True renewal builds gradually. Each week compounds your efforts, consistency turns signals into structure.

THE TAKEAWAY

Peptides don't "fix" aging, they **retrain your body's repair system.** By restoring growth signals, energizing fibroblasts, and improving sleep quality, they address the root cause of visible aging, not just the symptom.

Peptides remind your body how to rebuild itself.
They turn skincare into cell care, from surface beauty to structural vitality.

Disclaimer: *This content is for educational purposes only and is not a substitute for medical advice. Always consult a qualified healthcare professional before starting any new peptide, supplement, or hormone protocol.*

THE BEAUTY SIGNALS: Peptides for Visible Change

Let's stay practical: start with **low-risk, high-reward** signals and build from there.

1) GHK-Cu (Copper Peptide)

What it does: Stimulates collagen and elastin production, enhances wound healing, supports hair follicle vitality, and evens skin tone.
How to use: Apply as a topical serum or cream, morning or night. Pair with gentle exfoliation and daily sunscreen for optimal results. For advanced users, systemic approaches may be explored under the supervision of a clinician.
What to expect: Smoother texture within 4–6 weeks; firmer, more lifted appearance by 8–12 weeks.

2) Epitalon (Sleep & Longevity Support)

What it does: Balances circadian rhythm, promotes cellular housekeeping, and may improve skin tone through deeper recovery and growth hormone regulation.
How to use: Use in defined cycles under medical guidance; prioritize consistent sleep hygiene for synergy.
What to expect: More restorative sleep within 1–2 weeks; subtle radiance and even tone with sustained use.

3) Thymosin Family Support (e.g., TA-1 Context)

What it does: Modulates immune response, reduces inflammation, and supports smoother recovery after skin stress, treatments, or procedures.
How to use: Typically used under clinician direction during times of immune or inflammatory stress.
What to expect: Improved resilience, reduced flare-ups, and faster post-procedure healing.

4) Hair-Focused Signaling (GHK-Cu Topical, PTD-DBM Blends, Supportive Routines)

What it does: Encourages follicles to remain in the anagen (growth) phase, strengthens the scalp environment, and promotes thicker, healthier strands.

How to use: Apply consistently to the scalp, pairing it with weekly gentle microneedling (once a week) and nutrient-rich meals (including iron, zinc, and protein).
What to expect: Noticeable fullness and reduced shedding within 6–8 weeks of consistent application.

SUPPORT: Nutrition That Builds Radiance

Skin is built in the kitchen, refined in the gym, and polished in your sleep.

Topicals matter, but the *raw materials* for glow come from your meals.

The Collagen + Elastin Menu

- **Protein:** 30–40 g per meal. Include glycine-rich foods like bone broth, collagen peptides, and lean meats.
- **Vitamin C:** Essential for collagen cross-linking. Load up on citrus, kiwi, peppers, and berries.
- **Omega-3s:** 2 g combined EPA/DHA daily to support calm, hydrated skin.
- **Zinc + Selenium:** Crucial for hair strength and immune balance. Find them in seafood, eggs, and a few Brazil nuts.
- **Polyphenols:** Found in berries, green tea, and olive oil, protect skin from oxidative stress.
- **Water + Minerals:** Hydration shows on your skin. Add electrolytes if you sweat or train regularly.

Sample Day: 30-Day Meal Plan Preview (Beauty Phase)

Breakfast: Collagen matcha latte + Greek yogurt bowl with kiwi, chia, and walnuts.
Lunch: Wild salmon salad with olive oil, tomatoes, cucumbers, and a squeeze of citrus.
Snack: Cottage cheese + pineapple + pumpkin seeds.
Dinner: Lemon-herb chicken with asparagus, quinoa, and parsley.
Evening: Herbal tea; close the kitchen 3 hours before bed to support deep sleep and nightly renewal.

TOPICALS THAT WORK: Without a 20-Step Routine

Keep it simple. Consistency beats clutter.

Morning (3–5 minutes)

1. Gentle cleanse to remove overnight buildup.
2. Vitamin C serum: brightens and supports collagen.
3. GHK-Cu serum: apply a thin layer.
4. Moisturizer: Choose a ceramide-rich formula if your skin is dry.
5. Broad-spectrum sunscreen: protects against UV damage.

Evening (5–7 minutes)

1. Cleanse.
2. Gentle acid exfoliant 2–3×/week (lactic or mandelic) to support cell turnover.
3. GHK-Cu or peptide cream alternate nights with retinoid use.
4. Retinoid 2–4×/week as tolerated (avoid combining with strong acids most nights).
5. Moisturizer; add an occlusive layer if the skin is dry.

PRO TIP

If your skin is sensitive or reactive, introduce only one new product at a time and track results in your Journal. Calm, steady progress is the goal, not daily experimentation.

Hair Health: From Scalp Signals to Strong Strands

Thicker, stronger hair starts at the follicle. Healthy signals and a supportive scalp environment set the stage for visible results.

Signals & Supports

- **Topical GHK-Cu:** Boosts follicle vitality. Pair with gentle dermal rolling (0.5 mm) once weekly for optimal absorption.
- **PTD-DBM Blends (Professional Guidance):** Supports longer growth phases. Follow instructions carefully with clinician oversight.

- **Nutrition:** Prioritize protein, zinc, iron (if deficient), biotin from whole foods, and omega-3 fatty acids for follicle strength.
- **Stress & Sleep Management:** Cortisol spikes push follicles into rest. Maintain nightly routines and 7–9 hours of sleep to protect growth.
- **Gentle Hair Care:** Avoid tight hairstyles and high-heat tools. Use silk or satin pillowcases to reduce friction and breakage.

Track What Matters (Journal)

- Weekly shed count estimate
- Scalp comfort and sensitivity
- Bi-weekly photos under consistent lighting

TIP

Hair growth is slow, but consistent signaling, nutrition, and stress management compound over time. Track progress to stay motivated and catch early improvements.

The Beauty Timeline: What Realistic Progress Looks Like

Timeframe	Skin	Hair	What to Do
Weeks 1–2	Noticeable sleep glow; less morning puffiness	Scalp feels calmer	Nail the basics: cleanse, SPF, nightly wind-down, hydration
Weeks 3–4	Texture smoother; fine lines softer	Shed rate steadies	Add gentle exfoliation; keep protein intake high

Weeks 6–8	Firmer look; more even tone	Early fullness at hairline	Maintain signaling routines; avoid switching products too frequently
Weeks 10–12	Visible radiance; makeup sits better	Noticeable density in photos	Consider a maintenance block or targeted upgrades for continued improvement

REMEMBER

Light, consistent habits compound over time. Celebrate subtle wins, they accelerate bigger transformations.

Mini Story: "Glow Without the Grind"

Rina, 41, worked night shifts and felt like her natural glow had disappeared. She simplified her routine: GHK-Cu serum in the mornings, retinoid three times a week, sunscreen every day, a collagen matcha latte at breakfast, and a consistent lights-out routine at 10:30 PM on her days off.

After eight weeks, she wrote in her journal, "Makeup finally looks like an option, not a necessity." Her coworkers noticed the change before she did, a classic reminder that progress often shows up externally before we recognize it ourselves.

Takeaway: Consistency, simplicity, and aligning your lifestyle with your skin signals can create visible results without overwhelming routines.

Procedures, Peptides, and Recovery

If you choose in-office treatments like microneedling, lasers, or chemical peels, peptides can support a faster and smoother recovery when used in coordination with your professional.

Before Treatment:

- Hydrate thoroughly.
- Increase vitamin C intake through food to support collagen synthesis.
- Pause potent retinoids or exfoliating actives as advised.

After Treatment:

- Apply topical GHK-Cu to aid tissue repair and support fibroblast activity.
- Avoid harsh acids or retinoids until the skin is fully healed.

Sleep & Recovery:

- Prioritize 7–9 hours in a cool, dark room; journaling helps track patterns and quality.

Sun Protection:

- New collagen is vulnerable: use broad-spectrum sunscreen diligently.

Guiding Principle:

Your goal is **minimal irritation, maximal repair**. Patience and alignment with your body's natural repair signals ensure treatments amplify results without setbacks.

Hormone Context for Skin & Hair

Shifts in estrogen and progesterone influence skin thickness, moisture, and elasticity, while androgens affect oil production and hair patterns. Sudden dryness, sensitivity, or breakouts are often caused by hormonal fluctuations rather than product-related issues. Peptides can enhance repair and regeneration, but aligning sleep, nutrition, stress management, and professional guidance creates the optimal canvas for beauty signals to work.

Signs to watch with your clinician:

- Abrupt hair shedding
- Irregular cycles

- Hot flashes or night sweats
- Persistent cystic breakouts after 35

The Beauty Stack

1. Skin Glow Starter

- **Signals:** Topical GHK-Cu (AM or PM); sleep-support protocol (Epitalon cycle per guidance)
- **Support:** Vitamin C serum (AM), retinoid (PM 2–4×/week), SPF daily
- **Nutrition:** 30–40 g protein per meal + collagen scoop; berries daily
- **Timeline:** Texture improves in 3–4 weeks; firmness noticeable by 8–12 weeks

2. Hair Vitality Starter

- **Signals:** Scalp GHK-Cu + weekly dermal rolling; optional PTD-DBM blends with professional guidance
- **Support:** Zinc-rich foods, omega-3s, iron if low, gentle shampoo routine
- **Timeline:** Shed stabilizes by week 4; visible density by weeks 10–12

3. Even-Tone & Calm

- **Signals:** GHK-Cu + niacinamide; immune-tone support with guidance during flare seasons
- **Support:** Fragrance-free routine, patch test new products, consistent sun protection
- **Timeline:** Redness calms in 2–4 weeks; tone evens by 6–8 weeks

PRO TIP

The comprehensive 210 Stacks Guide organizes every combo by goal, enabling you to build efficient, goal-driven stacks with clear synergy and minimal overlap.

Sleep: The Ultimate Beauty Multiplier

No topical serum or supplement can rival the benefits of high-quality sleep. During deep sleep, growth hormone surges, collagen synthesis ramps up, and the glymphatic system clears toxins that dull your skin and mind. Think of your nighttime ritual as a full-body beauty routine: every cue you create signals your body to repair, rebuild, and refresh.

If you improve only **one variable this month**, make it your sleep.

Nighttime Wind-Down Checklist

- **Kitchen closed:** Finish eating at least 3 hours before bed
- **Screens off:** Turn off devices 60 minutes before lights-out
- **Gentle stretch or warm shower:** Relax muscles, reduce tension
- **Journaling:** Write 5 gratitude lines + 3 priorities for tomorrow
- **Sleep environment:** Keep room cool, dark, and quiet

TIP

Pair your ritual with peptides like Epitalon or CJC-1295 + Ipamorelin to amplify nighttime repair and visible beauty outcomes. Consistency here compounds every other effort in your routine.

Frequently Asked Questions

Q: Can I use GHK-Cu with a retinoid?

A: Yes, many people alternate them, copper peptide one night, retinoid another. If you layer, apply GHK-Cu first in a thin layer, then moisturizer. Always patch test and adjust based on comfort.

Q: What if I break out with new products?

A: Simplify and isolate variables. Stop all activities, reintroduce one at a time, and track reactions. Consider stress, sleep, and nutrition, your skin reflects what's happening inside.

Q: How long should I cycle Epitalon?
A: Follow professional guidance and the conservative cycles outlined later. Prioritize sleep hygiene; peptides amplify recovery, but cannot replace healthy habits.

Q: Is microneedling safe at home?
A: Gentle dermal rolling (0.3–0.5 mm) can be safe if done correctly. Disinfect tools, avoid harsh chemicals for 24–48 hours, and apply soothing, hydrating products. For more comprehensive treatments, consult a professional.

Q: Can peptides replace sunscreen?
A: Absolutely not. Daily SPF protects your skin from new damage. Peptides help repair and regenerate, but sunscreen preserves your progress.

Deep Dive: How Collagen Is Built (So You Can Build More)

Collagen is a triple-helix protein made from amino acids, mostly glycine, proline, and hydroxyproline. Fibroblasts act as the construction crew, stitching these strands together. Vitamin C acts as the quality-control manager, cross-linking fibers to impart strength and resilience. Copper and manganese help enzymes stabilize the matrix, while hyaluronic acid acts like a sponge, retaining water between fibers to achieve plumpness and bounce.

When sleep is shallow or protein intake is low, the assembly line slows. High UV exposure, stress, or inflammation can cause existing fibers to fray faster than they are replaced.

Key Takeaways:

- **Eat for building blocks:** prioritize protein, collagen peptides, and vitamin C-rich foods.

- **Sleep for the assembly line:** deep, restorative sleep supports fibroblast activity and growth hormone signaling.
- **Signal for productivity:** peptides like GHK-Cu and CJC-1295 + Ipamorelin amplify repair messages.
- **Protect the finished product:** daily SPF, antioxidants, and gentle topical routines prevent premature breakdown.

Collagen isn't just a cosmetic target, it's a dynamic system. Nourish, signal, and protect it, and your skin, hair, nails, and connective tissue all benefit.

Sugar, Glycation, and the "Sticky" Skin Problem

Excess sugar can attach to proteins in a process called glycation, creating advanced glycation end products (AGEs) that stiffen collagen. Stiff collagen doesn't bounce or reflect light as well, it looks dull, less supple, and creases more easily.

You don't need to fear every carbohydrate. Instead, **anchor carbs around movement** and prioritize fiber-rich sources. If sweets slip in, **pair them with protein and take a walk** to reduce the impact on glycation. This isn't punishment; it's physics, your body simply responds to the chemistry of your meals.

Key Takeaways:

- Glycation stiffens collagen, dulls skin, and accelerates visible aging.
- Timing and pairing carbs with activity helps minimize negative effects.
- Fiber-rich foods, protein, and movement protect your collagen matrix naturally.

By understanding glycation, you can enjoy carbs strategically while maintaining a firm, radiant, and resilient skin.

Sun, Blue Light, and Smart Protection

UV exposure is the fastest accelerator of visible skin aging. **Daily sunscreen is non-negotiable**, but effective protection goes beyond SPF.

Smart Habits for Sun & Light Protection:

- **Sunglasses:** Reduce squinting to prevent etched lines around the eyes.
- **Seek shade:** Especially during midday hours when UV is strongest.
- **Choose mineral sunscreens:** Zinc-based formulas are peptide-friendly and gentle on skin.
- **Blue light awareness:** Screens emit less intense light than the sun, but prolonged exposure can disrupt sleep. Enable night-shift modes and avoid late-night scrolling, sleep is a critical beauty tool.

PRO TIP

On long days outdoors, reapply sunscreen using a brush-on mineral powder for even application. It maintains a matte finish and layers easily over makeup.

By combining sunscreen, making lifestyle adjustments, and practicing mindful screen use, you can protect collagen, prevent premature lines, and maximize the impact of your peptide and skincare routines.

Red Light, Heat, and Cold: Do They Help?

These tools can support skin, recovery, and circulation, but they are **enhancers, not essentials**. Prioritize sleep, nutrition, and peptide signaling first.

Red / Near-Infrared Light:

- May improve skin tone, texture, and healing when used consistently.
- Treat it as a supportive habit: have short sessions several times a week.

Sauna / Heat:

- Boosts circulation and can enhance skin clarity.
- Always hydrate and replace electrolytes after sessions.

Cold Rinse / Cool Showers:

- Brief cold exposure at the end of showers can reduce redness and support recovery after workouts.

Key Reminder: *If these practices interfere with sleep, nutrition, or training,* ***adjust your priorities accordingly****. Think of light, heat, and cold as optional boosters; use them to complement your foundation, not replace it.*

The Scalp Microbiome & Hair Density

Your scalp is a living ecosystem. Maintaining good health is crucial for preserving hair density and promoting growth. Harsh shampoos, overwashing, and tight hairstyles can disrupt the microbiome and reduce microcirculation, limiting follicle function.

Tips for a Healthy Scalp:

- Use a gentle cleanser suited for your hair type.
- Massage the scalp during washing to stimulate circulation.
- Avoid overly tight hairstyles that restrict blood flow.
- If using dry shampoo, clarify weekly to prevent buildup that can suffocate follicles.

Weekly Ritual:

1. 5-minute gentle scalp massage.
2. Shampoo using light pressure.
3. Cool rinse to close follicles.
4. Pat your hair dry gently.
5. Apply GHK-Cu serum to the scalp.
6. Let hair air-dry when possible to minimize heat damage.

Following this routine consistently creates a supportive environment for follicles, enhances hair density, and maximizes the effect of peptides like GHK-Cu.

Nails, Hands, and Neck: The Forgotten Giveaways

Hands and neck often reveal age faster than the face due to higher sun exposure and less consistent care. Extend your facial routine to these areas for visible results.

Skin Care Tips:

- Apply vitamin C, moisturizer, and a broad-spectrum SPF daily to your hands and neck.
- At night, use a light hand cream containing urea or lactic acid (gloves optional for better absorption).
- Apply a neck-friendly retinoid 1–2 times per week to support collagen and firmness.

Nail Care Tips:

- Ensure sufficient protein intake; 1 g per pound of goal body weight supports strong nails.
- Add a collagen supplement or powder if nails peel or split easily.
- Stay hydrated; water supports nail health from within.
- File nails in one direction only to help prevent splitting, and avoid aggressive buffing, which can thin and weaken the nail plate.

By treating hands, neck, and nails as extensions of your face, you maintain consistency in your anti-aging strategy and ensure visible vitality beyond the mirror.

Sensitive Skin & Rosacea: Calm First, Correct Second

If your skin flushes easily, burns, or reacts to acids, simplify your routine. Focus on repairing the barrier before adding corrective treatments.

Calm-First Routine:

- **Cleanse gently:** Avoid fragrance and harsh surfactants.
- **Signal:** Apply a peptide serum to support fibroblast activity and healing.
- **Moisturize:** Use a ceramide-rich cream to strengthen the barrier.
- **Protect:** Mineral SPF daily.
- **Hold off on retinoids and strong actives** until the skin is calm. Layering too many active ingredients on inflamed skin can exacerbate sensitivity and diminish the effectiveness of peptides.

Lifestyle & Journal Tracking:

- Note triggers such as spicy foods, alcohol, hot showers, or late-night intense workouts.
- Patterns reveal which adjustments help your skin stay calm, recover faster, and respond better to peptides.

A stable, resilient barrier amplifies the benefits of every signal, making your skin more receptive to repair and renewal.

Men's Skin vs Women's Skin: Practical Differences

Men and women share fundamental skin characteristics, but differences in thickness, oil production, and hormonal fluctuations create practical variations.

Men:

- Skin tends to be thicker and oilier.
- Daily shaving provides mild exfoliation but can also irritate.
- **Routine Suggestions:**
  - Hydrating gel cleanser
  - Niacinamide or vitamin C in the morning
  - GHK-Cu peptide serum at night
  - Fragrance-free balm after shaving
  - Mineral SPF daily

Women:

- Skin may become thinner and drier due to hormonal shifts, particularly after the mid-30s.
- **Routine Suggestions:**
  - Creamy cleanser
  - Peptide serum layered under moisturizer
  - Retinoid 2–4×/week, adjusted for tolerance
  - SPF with added hydrating ingredients

Universal Principles:

- Sleep, protein, hydration, and sunscreen are beneficial to everyone.
- Beyond that, routines should be personalized to individual skin needs, sensitivities, and lifestyle.

Procedure Prep & Recovery: Safety-First Checklist

Two Weeks Before:

- Hydrate well and maintain high protein intake.
- Keep your skincare routine consistent.
- Avoid introducing new actives that could irritate your skin.

One Week Before:

- Pause harsh peels, acids, or retinoids if advised by your clinician.
- Boost vitamin C from whole foods.
- Prioritize sleep and stress management.

Day Of Procedure:

- Arrive with clean skin, following all clinician instructions.

After Procedure:

- Apply topical GHK-Cu as recommended.
- Use sunscreen diligently; new collagen is vulnerable.
- Skip retinoids or strong acids until cleared
- Sleep on clean pillowcases.
- Avoid hot yoga, saunas, or intense heat for the advised period.

Tracking Progress:

- Take photos under the same lighting every two weeks.
- Others often notice improvements before you do. Visual tracking reinforces the effectiveness of your routine.

Beauty Budget: Spend Where It Works

Top Priorities (High ROI):

- **Sleep setup:** Blackout shades, cool room, and consistent wind-down routine.
- **Nutrition:** Protein, collagen, berries, and olive oil - real food fuels repair and glow.
- **Sunscreen:** Daily mineral SPF you actually enjoy using.
- **Peptide topical (GHK-Cu):** Apply consistently for maximum effect.
- **Retinoid:** Evidence-backed texture and tone support.

Secondary / Optional (If Budget Allows):

- Devices or in-office procedures are only used after fundamentals are in place.

Guiding Principle:

- Buy fewer, better products; use them daily.
- Track adherence and results in your Journal, it's the simplest, most effective beauty upgrade.

Common Mistakes (and Easy Fixes)

1. **Switching routines too often**
   - **Mistake:** Jumping to a new product or routine weekly.
   - **Fix:** Commit to 8–12 weeks and change only one variable at a time to see real results.
2. **Skipping SPF on cloudy days**
   - **Mistake:** Thinking UV rays aren't intense when it's overcast.
   - **Fix:** Apply sunscreen every morning, as UV rays can penetrate clouds.
3. **Over-exfoliating**
   - **Mistake:** Using acids or scrubs too frequently, which can irritate.
   - **Fix:** Limit chemical exfoliants to 1–3 times a week; avoid abrasive scrubs.
4. **Late-night snacking**
   - **Mistake:** Eating right before bed, disrupting sleep and repair.
   - **Fix:** Close the kitchen 2–3 hours before bed; your skin and hair thrive on deep sleep.
5. **Treating hair without nutrition**
   - **Mistake:** Focusing only on topicals or styling products.
   - **Fix:** Prioritize protein and minerals first, then add supportive scalp/topical signals.

Progress You Can Feel (Not Just See)

People often notice compliments before numbers. Jackets sit better on the shoulders, the foundation glides on more smoothly, and hair brushes with less fallout. Capture these wins in your Journal. Tiny signals add up to the big reveal: you look like you've been sleeping, laughing, and living well, because you have.

Challenge	Likely Cause	Try This
Persistent dullness	Low sleep, low vitamin C	Lights out 30–60 min earlier; add citrus daily
Random breakouts	Overlapping activities or stress	Simplify routine; add daily walks; hydrate consistently
Flaky skin	Over-exfoliation, dry air	Reduce acids; use a humidifier; layer ceramide moisturizer
Hair shedding spike	Stress, low iron, sudden diet changes	Check labs with clinician; increase protein; scalp massage
Redness after retinoid	Too frequent use, weak barrier	Reduce to 1–2×/week; layer with moisturizer

TIP

Maintain a kind and curious approach. Skin and hair are conversations, not contests. Track, adjust, and celebrate small wins, they compound into lasting results.

Mini Story: "The Neck Reveal"

Jordan, 56, had focused on facial skincare for years but avoided her neck after a previous reaction to a strong acid. She restarted with a gentler plan: daily cleanser, GHK-Cu serum, moisturizer, and mineral SPF; retinoid once weekly, gradually increasing to twice weekly.

By week 8, photos revealed a smoother texture and fewer rings. Her note in the Journal:
"It wasn't a dramatic day-to-day until it was. Now I notice it in every Zoom call."

Sustain: Make Beauty Automatic

Automation beats motivation. Keep your morning serum next to your toothbrush for easy access. Set a recurring calendar reminder for weekly scalp care. Prep collagen scoops in a jar with the coffee. Turn your wind-down into a ritual you look forward to: book, tea, breathwork, bed.

Consistency matters more than intensity: signals stay strong when habits are easy.

Beauty is more effortless when your brain and mood work in harmony. Next up: **Sleep, Energy & Mood Reset**; the chapter that shows how to achieve deep rest, steady energy, and calm focus, so every system, including your skin, continues to improve.

CHAPTER 7

SLEEP, ENERGY & MOOD RESET POWER: RECLAIM CALM, FOCUS & DEEP RECOVERY

The Most Underestimated Power Tool: Sleep

Sleep is the most underrated performance enhancer on Earth. It regulates hormones, hunger, mood, recovery, and motivation, yet it's the first habit most of us sacrifice when life gets busy.

After 35, deep sleep often starts to slip. You fall asleep easily but wake at 2 a.m. with your mind racing. You hit snooze one too many times, drag through mornings that once felt effortless, and rely on caffeine to survive the day. Before long, fatigue feels "normal," cravings return, and focus fades even when you're eating clean and working out.

That's not a weakness. It's biology adapting to stress and time.
When your sleep rhythm breaks:

- Growth hormone (GH) pulses shrink
- Recovery slows
- Inflammation rises

Every system peptides aim to optimize metabolism, repair, and renewal, depending on the foundation of deep, restorative sleep.
This chapter shows you how to:

- Reset your circadian rhythm
- Lower nighttime cortisol
- Activate the body's natural repair cycles

No peptide, workout, or nutrition plan can outperform a body ruled by exhaustion and stress chemistry.

When sleep returns, everything else starts working again, energy, focus, recovery, and joy.

Why Modern Life Wrecks Recovery

Blue-light exposure, late-night emails, caffeine past noon, and constant notifications all distort the body's master clock. Add hormonal shifts and nightly alcohol "wind-downs," and your circadian rhythm gets scrambled. Growth-hormone pulses flatten, cortisol spikes at the wrong times, and mood neurotransmitters lose rhythm.

The fix isn't sedation, it's **signal synchronization**: teaching your brain and body to trust the clock again.

The Power Wellness Sleep Formula

Element	Signal Type	Daily Action	Why It Matters
Light	Morning cue	Get 5–10 min outside within 30 min of waking	Anchors circadian rhythm
Movement	Metabolic cue	Walk or stretch mid-morning	Lowers cortisol
Protein Breakfast	Nutrient cue	30 g protein + complex carbs	Stabilizes glucose & neurotransmitters
Caffeine Cutoff	Chemical cue	Stop caffeine by 2 p.m.	Prevents interference with adenosine accumulation
Wind-down Ritual	Behavioral cue	Screens off one hour before bed; gentle stretch/breathing	Naturally raises melatonin
Sleep Stack	Peptide cue	DSIP + CJC/Ipamorelin at night	Deepens restorative sleep stages

Peptides That Reset Rest

1) DSIP: Delta Sleep Inducing Peptide

- **Role:** Balances sleep cycles, reduces nighttime cortisol, supports parasympathetic dominance.
- **When:** 30–60 min before bed on non-training nights.
- **Expected:** Fewer 2 a.m. wake-ups by week 2; calmer mornings.

2) Selank: The Anxiety Modulator

- **Role:** Stabilizes GABA and serotonin; improves focus without sedation.
- **When:** Morning micro-dose or pre-meeting during stress spikes.
- **Stack Tip:** Pairs well with Semax for balanced alertness.

3) Semax: Cognitive Clarity

- **Role:** Enhances BDNF (brain-derived neurotrophic factor) for learning and memory.
- **When:** Morning or early afternoon only.
- **Expected:** Improved concentration within days; mental fatigue declines by week 2.

***Note:** These peptides amplify healthy sleep and stress habits; they do **not** replace proper sleep hygiene, nutrition, or stress management.*

Nutrition for Neurotransmitters

Food is more than fuel, it's chemistry for mood and sleep. Adequate protein and key micronutrients provide the building blocks for serotonin, dopamine, and GABA, which help regulate focus, calm, and restorative sleep.

Core Nutrients & Sources

- **Tryptophan → Serotonin:** Turkey, eggs, pumpkin seeds.
- **Tyrosine → Dopamine:** Chicken, beef, fish, bananas.
- **Magnesium & Vitamin B6:** Leafy greens, nuts, avocado.
- **Omega-3s:** Fish oil supports anti-inflammatory balance.
- **Electrolytes:** Maintain nervous-system calm and signal efficiency.

Sample Evening Meal (Sleep Phase: 30-Day Plan Preview)

- **Salmon with spinach & quinoa** → high-quality protein + tryptophan.

- **Berries with Greek yogurt** → magnesium and antioxidants.
- **Chamomile tea** → glycine and GABA support for calm and deeper sleep.

PRO TIPS

- Avoid heavy meals within 3 hours of bedtime, as late digestion can blunt growth hormone release.
- Pair nutrition with a consistent wind-down routine to maximize neurotransmitter support.

Training Timing & Sleep

Exercise is a powerful **zeitgeber, a signal** that helps set your internal clock. Timing your workouts strategically can enhance both energy and restorative sleep:

- **Morning / Early Day Workouts:** Boost alertness, stabilize circadian rhythm, and prime daytime metabolism.
- **Evening Workouts:** Can raise core body temperature and delay sleep onset. If evenings are your only option:
    - Finish at least **3 hours before going to bed**.
    - Include a **slow cool-down** with stretching and deep breathing.
    - Optional: **5-minute cold rinse or contrast shower** to signal relaxation and aid temperature drop for sleep.

Takeaway: Align your workouts with your sleep goals, as exercise supports your energy and recovery; however, timing is crucial for achieving deep, restorative rest.

Caffeine, Alcohol, and Hidden Sleep Thieves

- **Caffeine:** Half-life ~6 hours. That 2 p.m. latte can still impact your 10 p.m. sleep. Aim to **cut caffeine by early afternoon**.
- **Alcohol:** Sedates initially but **disrupts REM cycles**, leading to fragmented rest. Avoid drinking **within 3 hours of bedtime**.
- **Screens & Blue Light:** Suppresses melatonin up to 50%. Use **warm filters**, dim lighting, or **audio-only content** after 9 p.m.

- **Late Exercise:** High-intensity training raises adrenaline and core temperature. **Add extra wind-down time** if you train in the evening.

Action Step: Track caffeine, alcohol, screen time, and evening workouts for **one week in your Journal**. Identify patterns and adjust habits for deeper, restorative sleep.

Morning Momentum: How You Wake Determines How You Sleep

Sleep is a **24-hour cycle**, and how you start your day sets the tone for restorative rest at night.

Power AM Routine:

1. **Sunlight Exposure:** Open curtains immediately; light signals your brain that the day has begun.
2. **Hydration:** Drink water with electrolytes before your coffee to jumpstart circulation.
3. **Protein Breakfast:** Eat within 60 minutes to stabilize glucose and support neurotransmitters.
4. **Movement:** Move for ≥10 minutes, stretch, walk, or exercise outdoors if possible.
5. **Gratitude Journal:** Write a quick note to prime dopamine pathways and enhance mood.

Why It Matters: By syncing your morning cues with natural light, nutrition, and movement, your **melatonin signal rises faster in the evening**, helping you fall asleep more easily and sleep more deeply.

Stress & Cortisol Rhythm

Chronic stress can flatten your natural cortisol curve, too high at night, too low in the morning.

Symptoms: Wired but tired evenings, mid-day crashes, sugar cravings, and anxiety.

Peptides like **Selank** can help rebalance stress signaling, but daily **parasympathetic training** (governs rest, recovery, digestion and repair) is essential to restore your body's natural rhythm.

Parasympathetic Tools:

- **Breathing Exercises:** 4-7-8 or box breathing before bed to calm the nervous system.
- **Journaling:** Five-minute reflection to release mental tension.
- **Gentle Movement:** Short walks after meals to activate relaxation pathways.
- **Consistent Sleep Schedule:** Go to bed and wake up within a 30-minute window daily.

Pro Tip: 4-7-8 breathing is one of the fastest ways to activate your parasympathetic nervous system. Inhale for 4 seconds, hold for 7 seconds, and exhale for 8 seconds. The long, slow exhale signals your body to relax, lowers tension, and prepares you for deeper sleep.

Why It Matters: Every signal of safety lowers adrenal output, reopens healing pathways, and supports fat loss, muscle growth, and overall recovery.

Mini Story: "From Insomnia to Insight"

Eric, 47, was surviving on five hours of sleep most nights and leaning on energy drinks to get through the day. He began the **Power Sleep Stack**, consisting of **DSIP and CJC/Ipamorelin at night,** and **Selank during the day**, while consistently logging his sleep in his Journal.

- **Week 2:** First unbroken six hours of sleep.
- **Week 4:** 7½ hours, no afternoon crash.

Eric reflected, "My mood lifted before my energy did. That's when I knew I was healing." The mirror confirmed it: less facial bloating, brighter eyes, and stronger workouts.

Evening Ritual Template (Download Preview)

Wind-Down Block: 30 minutes

- **Warm shower** → relax muscles and signal the body it's time to wind down.
- **Dim lights** to ~50% brightness.

- **Chamomile tea + collagen scoop** → hydration + amino acids for overnight repair.
- **Breathing track or guided prayer** → calm the nervous system.
- **Bedtime** → aim for 10:00 p.m. window.
- **Journal Prompt:**
- Record bedtime, wake time, and sleep quality (scale 1–10).
- Review your routine after one week to spot patterns and optimize it.

Mood Reset & Cognitive Clarity

Energy isn't just physical, it's emotional and cognitive. Balanced neurotransmitters (dopamine, serotonin, acetylcholine) help you feel motivated, focused, and calm.

Mood Stack Example:

Morning

- Semax (as directed)
- Omega-3 supplement
- 10–15 min sunlight walk → natural circadian cue

Afternoon

- Protein-rich snack
- Hydration (water or electrolyte beverage)

Evening

- Selank (0.1 ml nasal)
- Gratitude journaling
- 5–10 min breathwork or relaxation practice

Expected Results:

- By week 2: clearer thinking, steady energy, and reduced mental fatigue.
- Supports mood, focus, and overall cognitive clarity when paired with sleep hygiene and nutrition.

Common Sleep Blockers & Quick Fixes

Problem	Likely Cause	Quick Reset
Can't fall asleep	Late screens, caffeine	Use blue-light filters; stop caffeine by 2 p.m.
Wake at 2–3 a.m.	Low glycogen, high stress	Add evening protein; 5–10 min breathing or meditation
Groggy mornings	Irregular wake time	Set the same alarm 7 days/week; morning sunlight exposure
Night sweats	Hormone shifts	Cool room; cotton sheets; check thyroid if persistent
Racing mind	Cortisol surge	DSIP before bed; 4-7-8 or box breathing

TIP

Track your sleep and triggers in a Journal for 1–2 weeks. Patterns reveal which reset strategies work best for you.

Hormones & Neurochemistry After 35

As we age, key hormones shift:

- **Estrogen & Progesterone (Women):** Progesterone promotes calm sleep; its decline can lead to increased nighttime anxiety.
- **Testosterone (Men & Women):** Supports energy, mood, and deep restorative sleep.
- **Growth Hormone (GH):** Declines in GH lead to reduced slow-wave sleep, which limits recovery and tissue repair.

Key Insight: Peptides can enhance hormone signaling and reset rhythms, but they cannot override chaotic lifestyle habits. Sleep, stress management, and nutrition remain essential.

Action: If you experience persistent fatigue, disrupted sleep, or hormonal symptoms, consider getting lab tests and consulting with a functional clinician. Combining hormonal balance with peptides maximizes restorative sleep, think "sleep of your twenties with the wisdom of your forties."

The Energy Equation

Energy = Mitochondria × Efficiency

Energy isn't created from caffeine or sheer willpower, it's produced at the cellular level. Your mitochondria, tiny engines in every cell, convert oxygen and nutrients into ATP, the molecule that powers movement, thought, and repair. When those engines run efficiently, life feels lighter: focus is steadier, recovery is faster, and drive lasts longer.

1. Train the Engines, Don't Drain Them

- Short, moderate sessions of **Zone 2 cardio** (60–70% of maximum heart rate) teach mitochondria to burn fuel more efficiently.
- Zone-2 expands **mitochondrial density**: more engines per cell, more endurance per effort.
- **Consistency beats intensity:** 30 minutes, three times per week outperforms sporadic, exhausting workouts.

2. Signal Smarter with Peptides

- **Semax** enhances brain oxygen use by increasing **BDNF**, improving mitochondrial ATP production in both muscle and neural tissue.
- Fine-tunes alertness and stamina without overstimulation.
- Best used during focus-heavy phases or demanding training blocks to sustain energy naturally.

3. Protect Cellular Output

- **Nutrients:** CoQ10, magnesium, and carnitine support ATP synthesis.
- **Breathing:** Nasal or diaphragmatic patterns during exercise improve oxygen delivery.
- **Recovery:** Light post-training movement and nutrient intake keep energy pathways open.

4. Skip the Quick Fix

- Stimulants borrow energy from tomorrow, creating crashes.
- Optimized mitochondria produce energy on demand, no repayment required.
- Efficient energy systems sharpen focus, reduce fatigue, and naturally stabilize mood.

Bottom Line

Energy isn't about pushing harder, it's about running cleaner.

- **Train the mitochondria** with consistent, moderate movement.
- **Signal intelligently** with peptides like Semax.
- **Feed the engines** with the raw materials they need: protein, micronutrients, and oxygen.

Do this consistently, and energy stops being a struggle, it becomes your baseline. Efficient cells = effortless power.

Educational purposes only. Consult a qualified professional before starting peptide or supplement protocols.

Mini Story: "Calm Focus at Last"

Nina, 52, juggled a full-time job and caring for aging parents. She started using Selank in the mornings and DSIP at night. Within six weeks, her Journal showed sleep scores steadily rising from 4 to 8.

Her note: *"I stopped snapping at small things. My energy didn't spike, it stabilized."*

That's real power: calm focus without fatigue.

Checklist: Your 14-Day Sleep Reboot

- Morning light exposure within 30 minutes of waking
- Caffeine cutoff by 2 p.m.
- Include protein in every meal
- Screens off 1 hour before bed
- DSIP nightly (weeks 1–2)
- Selank for stress control AM/PM

- Journal sleep and mood daily

Repeat this consistently for 14 days and review your patterns. You'll notice energy returning, even before changes in weight, skin, or performance appear.

With nighttime recovery restored and daytime performance stabilized, you're ready to fortify defense and longevity. Next up: Immune & Longevity Power, extending cellular repair signals to resilience, vitality, and lifespan.

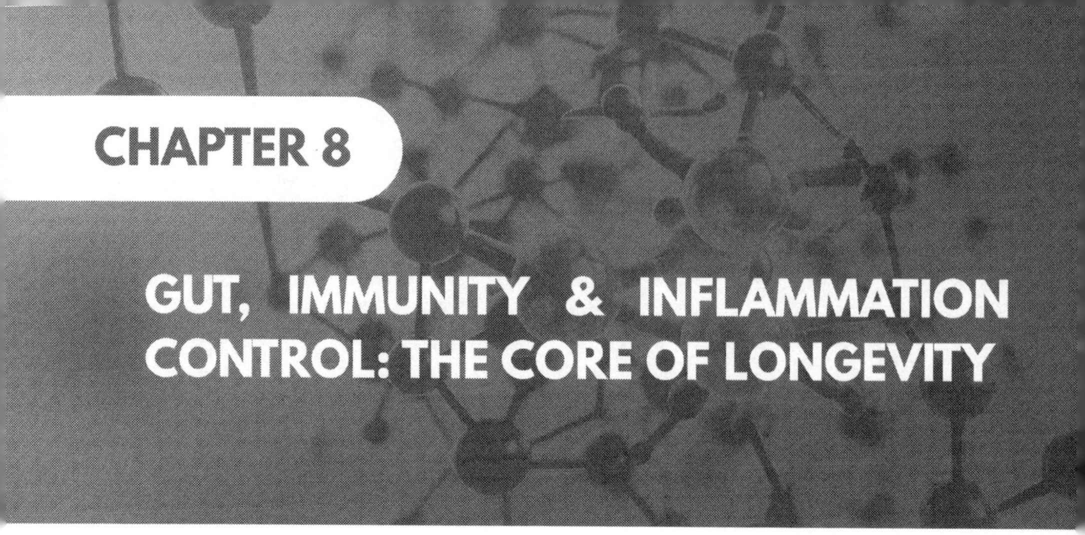

CHAPTER 8

GUT, IMMUNITY & INFLAMMATION CONTROL: THE CORE OF LONGEVITY

If your gut isn't happy, nothing else in your body runs smoothly.

After 35, digestion and immune strength often decline together, bloating sets in, energy levels dip, skin becomes dull, and inflammation appears in unexpected places, including joints, mood, and even sleep.

This isn't random. Your gut is the command center for nearly 70% of your immune system and your most powerful regulator of inflammation. When gut communication breaks down, the body stops repairing and starts reacting.

This chapter shows how to calm that inner fire so every peptide, nutrient, and recovery habit you've built so far can finally work at full strength.

When you restore gut balance, you upgrade metabolism, immunity, and longevity in one coordinated move.

The Gut–Immune Axis in Plain English

Imagine your gut lining as a **24-hour security system.** Every meal brings both nutrients and potential irritants. The intestinal wall decides what enters your bloodstream and what gets rejected. When the lining becomes damaged due to stress, antibiotics, alcohol, sugar, or a low-fiber diet, **tiny gaps** open between cells. Immune cells rush in to defend you, releasing cytokines, the **chemical sparks of inflammation.**

In the short term, this response protects you. Long-term, it creates **systemic noise**, the background buzz of inflammation that manifests as joint stiffness, bloating, mood dips, or brain fog. These are not "just signs of aging." They're signals that communication has broken down.

The goal isn't to silence your immune system, it's to **teach it to whisper again.** That process starts with **restoring the gut barrier** and **retraining the immune response** to react appropriately, not excessively.

Peptides That Soothe and Rebuild

BPC-157: The Tissue Healer

Derived from natural gastric proteins, **BPC-157** signals the body to rebuild damaged intestinal tissue. It boosts blood flow, supports ulcer healing, and strengthens the gut barrier for improved nutrient absorption. Within weeks, most users notice less bloating, steadier digestion, and faster workout recovery.

- **Cycle:** 250–500 mcg daily for 4–8 weeks
- **Synergy:** Combine with collagen and omega-3 fats
- **Journal Cue:** Track morning bloating (0–10) and note digestion ease

KPV: The Inflammation Switch-Off

A calming fragment of alpha-MSH, **KPV** acts like an internal fire extinguisher.
It suppresses **NF-κB**, the body's master inflammatory signal, helping soothe IBS, eczema, and post-training soreness. Both topical and oral forms work systemically.

- **Cycle:** 250 mcg 1–2× daily for 2–6 weeks
- **Pairing:** Combine with BPC-157 for gut + skin synergy
- **Expected:** Reduced redness, smoother digestion, calmer joints

TB-500: The Repair Accelerator

A fragment of **Thymosin Beta-4**, **TB-500** enhances cell formation and tissue regeneration by stimulating actin and new blood vessel growth. It complements BPC-157 by improving oxygen delivery and speeding recovery in muscles, joints, and organs.

- **Cycle:** 2–5 mg weekly for 4–6 weeks
- **Support:** Hydration + magnesium
- **Stack Cue:** Combine BPC + TB for full-body tissue regeneration

GLP-2 Analogs: The Absorption Optimizers

Emerging **GLP-2** peptides help strengthen the gut lining and restore nutrient absorption, particularly after prolonged periods of dieting, illness, or stress. They rebuild microvilli, the tiny, nutrient-absorbing "fingers" of the intestinal wall, which improves energy and reduces post-meal crashes.

- **Frequency:** Every other day or as directed by your clinician
- **Effect:** Better nutrient uptake, steadier energy, and smoother digestion

Nutrition for Gut Calm and Immune Strength

Peptides repair from within, but the food we consume determines whether that repair lasts.

To keep inflammation low and absorption high, build your meals around this **Power Plate for Inflammation Control.**

Component	Function	Examples
Protein (Repair)	Builds enzymes and immune cells	Fish, eggs, poultry, collagen
Color (Antioxidant)	Neutralizes inflammation	Berries, spinach, peppers
Fiber (Microbiome)	Feeds beneficial bacteria	Oats, beans, chia, artichokes
Fat (Hormone Support)	Regulates immune response	Olive oil, avocado, nuts
Spices (Defense)	Natural anti-inflammatories	Turmeric, ginger, garlic

Simple Rule:
Half your plate color + one palm protein + two tablespoons healthy fat + one fist starch (if training).

Sample Day: Gut Phase (30-Day Plan Preview)

Breakfast: Greek yogurt + berries + chia + collagen
Lunch: Salmon + quinoa + broccoli + olive oil
Snack: Green tea + walnuts
Dinner: Chicken + sweet potato + spinach + garlic
Evening: Chamomile tea, kitchen closed 3 hours before bed

Microbiome 101: Your Internal Pharmacy

Your gut bacteria outnumber your human cells **ten to one.** They act like a built-in pharmacy, producing neurotransmitters, vitamins, and fat-burning molecules that keep your metabolism, mood, and immune system in sync. When antibiotics, chronic stress, or ultra-processed foods disrupt this ecosystem, the result is inflammation, fatigue, and brain fog.

How to Rebuild the Microbiome

- **Prebiotic fiber:** Veggies, beans, and oats feed your good bacteria.
- **Fermented foods:** Yogurt, kefir, and kimchi introduce new strains.
- **Probiotic cycles:** Use a 4–8 week on, 4 week off cycle to support diversity.
- **Polyphenols:** Berries, olive oil, and green tea, protect existing colonies.

Journal Prompt:

- Track energy and bloating after adding one new food.
- Improvement means balance is returning.

Stress, Sleep & the Inflammation Loop

Your gut has its own nervous system, known as the **enteric nervous system,** which communicates with your central nervous system through the **vagus nerve.**

When stress levels rise, digestion slows, stomach acid production decreases, and harmful bacteria multiply. That's why chronic anxiety or poor sleep can mimic food intolerance or trigger bloating and fatigue.

Reset the Loop

- **Slow breathing:** 3 minutes morning and night to activate the vagus nerve.
- **Morning sunlight:** Anchors your circadian rhythm and helps balance cortisol levels.
- **Meal timing:** Finish eating 2–3 hours before bed to ease overnight repair.
- **Peptide support:** Microdoses of *Selank* or *DSIP* can help stabilize sleep patterns when stress levels are high.

Sleep is your most natural anti-inflammatory therapy, protecting you like medicine.

Anti-Inflammatory Lifestyle Checklist

- **Hydrate:** At least ½ your body weight (lbs) in ounces daily
- **Move daily:** 8–10K steps or light activity
- **Build strength:** Train 2–3× per week
- **Contrast therapy:** Sauna or cool rinse if available
- **Moderate indulgence:** Alcohol and sugar kept rare
- **Mood medicine:** Laugh often, get sunlight every day

Inflammation thrives on chaos and starves it.

Peptide Power Stack Examples: Gut & Inflammation

Stack	Peptides	Cycle	Support	Journal Focus
Gut Repair Stack	BPC-157 + KPV	8 wks	Collagen + fiber + probiotic	Bloating & energy

Inflammation Reset	BPC-157 + TB-500	6 wks	Turmeric + omega-3	Pain & mobility
Immune Calm Stack	TA-1 + KPV	6 wks	Sleep + vitamin D	Sick days per month
Recovery Stack	BPC-157 + GHK-Cu	6 wks	Protein + hydration	Skin clarity & digestive ease

The Inflammation Gauge: Track What Matters

Skip the guesswork.
Use this five-point self-check weekly in your Journal to spot trends before they turn into setbacks.

Signal	1 (Low)	5 (Moderate)	10 (High)	Signal
Morning stiffness	None	Noticeable	Painful	Morning stiffness
Bloating	Flat	Mild	Constant	Bloating
Energy	High	Midday dip	Crash	Energy
Mood	Calm	Irritable	Anxious	Mood
Sleep	Deep	Interrupted	Restless	Sleep

Inflammation Index:
Add your five scores → divide by 5.

If your Index stays ≥6 for two weeks:
Adjust your *food* and *stress* patterns before changing your stack.

Real-World Story: “From Inflamed to Energized”

Maria, 47, struggled with daily bloating, joint aches, and brain fog. She started a simple **BPC-157 + KPV stack**, shifted to a **Mediterranean-style plate**, and tracked her **Inflammation Index** weekly.

After six weeks, her score dropped from **8 → 3**. Her journal entry captured the shift:
"I don't feel 'on a program' anymore, my body finally feels quiet."

Mindset: Healing From the Inside Out

Your gut isn't fragile, it's **adaptable**. Every symptom you experience is a signal asking for clearer communication. Peptides help **translate** that language, but your habits **write the message**. Every time you **breathe slower, eat with focus, or keep consistent meals**, you tell your body it's safe, and safety is where true recovery begins.

Power Prompt:

- What single habit calms my system fastest?
- Do it twice a day for one week and observe the changes.

When inflammation subsides, **clarity returns**, both in the body and the mind. With your gut balanced and immune rhythm restored, you're ready for **precision**.

Next up: the **Stack Mastery Guide**, where you'll design your **personalized plan** inside the Power Wellness framework.

CHAPTER 9

STACK MASTERY GUIDE: BUILD YOUR CUSTOM PLAN WITH CONFIDENCE

Knowledge becomes power the moment you turn it into motion. You already understand how peptides spark repair, how nutrition fuels that spark, and how consistency turns small actions into lasting transformation. Now it's time to connect the dots. This chapter serves as your blueprint, the structure that transforms scattered effort into results you can see and feel. You don't need 20 peptides; you need purpose, precision, and the right combinations speaking your body's language. Think of stacking like music. Every peptide plays its part, and when the rhythm is correct, your body performs like a symphony.

The Power Wellness Stacking Philosophy

1. **Signal First:** Peptides are instruction sets. Select only those aligned with your core goal: fat loss, recovery, beauty, or longevity.
2. **Support Second:** Nutrition, hydration, sleep, and movement amplify every signal. Without them, peptides whisper into noise.
3. **Simplify Third:** Two to three synergistic peptides consistently outperform six competing ones.
4. **Cycle Fourth:** Most protocols are most effective in 8–12 week blocks, followed by a rest period.
5. **Track Always:** Your Journal is your lab. Log mood, energy, sleep, and visual progress weekly to see what truly works.

Safety First: Stack Hierarchy

Before building your stack, review the hierarchy and progress only when the previous tier is stable and reliable.

Tier	Purpose	Peptide Examples	Duration
Foundation	Restore baseline recovery & sleep	CJC-1295 + Ipamorelin, DSIP	8–12 weeks
Functional	Target specific tissues (fat, muscle, joints)	AOD-9604, BPC-157, TB-500	6–12 weeks
Enhancement	Optimize cognitive, beauty, or immune signals	Semax, GHK-Cu, TA-1	4–8 weeks
Longevity	Support cellular aging & repair	Epitalon cycle blocks	10–20 days × quarter

TIP

Only move to the next tier once the previous tier feels stable. Stability ensures that signals are built on a solid foundation, rather than competing or overwhelming one another.

How to Choose Your Goal Stack

- **Define Outcome** Identify the area that frustrates you most right now: energy, pain, fat loss, skin clarity, or recovery.
- **Match Peptide to Outcome** Refer to the Stacks PDF to see which peptides align with your goal.
- **Select Cycle Length** Most protocols: 8–12 weeks. Longevity peptides often run shorter cycles (10–20 days per quarter).

- **Decide Frequency**
  - Daily: Growth hormone or healing peptides
  - 1–2× per week: Immune support peptides
- **Log Data** Record mood, energy, sleep, and visual changes in your Journal, your entries are your proof of progress.

Rule of Three: *Use no more than three active signals at a time to avoid competing instructions.*

Quick-Reference Stack Table

Goal	Core Peptides	Cycle	Key Support	Journal Focus
Fat Loss Accelerator	CJC-1295 + Ipamorelin + AOD-9604	12 weeks	Protein + steps + sleep	Weight & energy curve
Lean Muscle Builder	CJC-1295 + Ipamorelin + BPC-157	10 weeks	Strength training	Recovery score
Joint Repair Stack	BPC-157 + TB-500	8 weeks	Mobility + omega-3s	Pain 0–10 rating
Beauty & Glow	GHK-Cu (topical) + Epitalon	8 weeks	Collagen + sleep	Skin photos
Sleep & Calm	DSIP + Selank	4 weeks	Wind-down ritual	Sleep hours
Immune Reset	TA-1 + Epitalon	6 weeks	Vitamin D + zinc	Energy stability
Longevity Maintenance	Epitalon (quarterly)	10–20 days	Zone-2 cardio	Resting HR trend

Timing & Injection Log

Day	Peptide / Dose	Time	Injection Site	Sleep (hrs)	Energy (1–10)
Mon	CJC + Ipamorelin	10 PM	Abdomen	7.5	8
Tue	AOD-9604	7 AM	Abdomen	8	9
Wed	BPC-157	8 AM	Thigh	7	8
Thu	CJC + Ipamorelin	10 PM	Abdomen	7.5	8
Fri	Rest Day	—	—	8	9

Stack Combos to Avoid

- **Multiple GH releasers at once** → May cause fatigue, water retention, or hormone imbalance.
- **Overlapping immune peptides** (e.g., TA-1 + LL-37 + long-term TB-500) → Risk of overstimulation or dysregulated immune response.
- **Neglecting foundation habits** → Peptides cannot compensate for poor sleep, nutrition, or stress management.
- **Skipping cycle breaks** → Always cycle off 8–12 weeks to reset receptors and avoid tolerance.

PRO TIP

Focus on signal + support + cycle discipline. Fewer, targeted peptides produce better results than stacking everything at once. Always consult a clinician.

When to Upgrade a Stack

Consider upgrading or adjusting your stack when:

1. **Full Cycle Completed** – You've finished the recommended 8–12 week block.
2. **Stable Recovery & Energy** – Sleep scores and daily energy are consistently ≥ 8/10.
3. **Consistent Results** – Journal entries show stable weight, mood, and performance metrics.
4. **No Adverse Effects** – You've been free of side effects for at least 30 days.

Next Step: Add **one new peptide signal** or shift to a different goal-focused stack. Avoid multiple simultaneous changes to keep progress measurable.

Practical Cycle Calendar

Weeks 1–4:

- Establish your **foundation stack**.
- Log key metrics: sleep, energy, recovery, mood, and performance.

Weeks 5–8:

- Assess progress by evaluating sleep quality, recovery speed, and energy consistency.
- Adjust support habits (nutrition, hydration, movement) as needed.

Weeks 9–12:

- Peak cycle performance.
- Track measurable outcomes, such as strength, fat loss, skin, or joint improvements.

Weeks 13–14:

- **Deload phase**: Reduce intensity while maintaining key habits.
- Review journal notes and cycle performance.

Weeks 15–16:

- Reevaluate your goals and plan your **next cycle** based on the results you achieve.

Built-in reflection ensures progress is sustainable and measurable, preventing burnout or overstacking.

Mindset: From Protocol to Practice

The ultimate goal is **autonomy**. After this chapter, you'll know how to plan safely, confidently, and without guesswork. Remember:

- **You are the experiment, not the lab rat.** Let your data guide adjustments.
- **Simplicity scales.** Stacks that fit your life are the ones you'll actually maintain.
- **Consistency beats complexity.** Results follow steady, repeatable habits, not complicated routines.

With each cycle you complete, you build **self-trust**, the real secret behind Peptide Power.

You've rebuilt communication inside your body: cells signal clearly, inflammation quiets, and energy flows. Now, the real work begins: **keeping it that way.**

Lasting change doesn't come from perfection, it comes from **rhythm**. When movement, meals, mindset, and rest run on autopilot, health stops feeling like effort and starts feeling like **identity**.

The next chapter presents a **friction-free framework** to protect your progress, amplify your results, and make wellness automatic - **no willpower required.**

CHAPTER 10

THE POWER LIFESTYLE SYSTEM: MAKE RESULTS AUTOMATIC

You've rebuilt the conversation inside your body, fat loss launched, muscle strengthened, pain calmed, skin brighter, sleep deeper, mood steadier, and immunity smarter. Now comes what most programs skip: turning results into a rhythm so you don't slide back when life gets loud.

This chapter gives you a friction-proof operating system that works in real life without living like a monk or turning wellness into a full-time job.

At the heart of it is a repeatable loop you can run for years:

Stabilize → Build → Peak → Deload → Sustain

- Each phase lasts weeks, not months.
- Each has clear inputs (habits + stacks) and outputs (metrics) so you always know if you're on track.

This chapter focuses on how the loop works and how to live inside it. The day-by-day 30-day plan appears later and does not repeat what's covered here.

The Five-Phase Loop

Stabilize (≈ 2 weeks)

Purpose: Create predictable days so recovery and appetite settle.

Signals: Keep it minimal. If you just finished a high-output cycle, pause new additions and continue only baseline sleep support if used.

Habits you can automate in three days:

- Morning light within 30 minutes of waking
- Protein at breakfast (30–40 g)
- 8–10k steps across the day (split walks count)
- Screen-off hour before bed; kitchen closed 3 hours before bed

Metrics: Sleep hours, morning energy (1–10), waist
Outcome: Steady, not heroic. This steadiness is your launchpad.

Build (≈ 4 weeks)

Purpose: Pick one clear goal (fat loss, muscle, skin, or joint repair) and align your inputs.
Signals: Choose one goal-based starter stack. No extras yet.
Training: 3–4 resistance sessions or 2 resistance + 2 cardio depending on the goal
Nutrition: Protein-anchored meals timed around movement; hydration consistent
Metrics: Weekly progress photos, training log, morning energy, sleep quality
Outcome: Predictable momentum, you can point to what improved and why

Peak (≈ 2–4 weeks)

Purpose: Harvest the best results with tight execution without burnout
Signals: Continue the same stack; consider one supportive add-on only if sleep and energy average ≥ 8/10 for two weeks
Training: Progressive overload for strength or gently increase step target for fat loss; avoid stacking HIIT every day
Recovery: Keep deload planned. A great peak ends clean, not exhausted
Metrics: Journal your Best-Day pattern (bedtime, meals, movement) and replicate
Outcome: Maximum results without sacrifice

Deload (≈ 1–2 weeks)

Purpose: Reset receptors and nervous system so you can keep progressing

Signals: Reduce or pause goal-specific peptides; keep sleep/repair support if desired
Training: Lower volume and intensity by ~30–40%; keep technique sharp
Nutrition: Return to maintenance calories with high protein; emphasize micronutrients
Metrics: Mood steadiness, resting heart rate on waking, perceived recovery
Outcome: Finish fresher than you started, ready to train again

Sustain (≈ 4+ weeks)

Purpose: Convert results into identity
Signals: Minimal: often only sleep support or topical beauty routine
Training: 2–3 strength sessions, daily walks, small mobility blocks
Nutrition: Maintainable meals that match your schedule; batch-cook proteins on the weekend
Metrics: Once-weekly waist and photo check-in; nothing obsessive
Outcome: Progress holds without willpower. When life spikes, you don't crash, you flex

Make It Automatic: The Four Default Days

High performers don't plan every hour, they run **defaults**. Put these in your calendar notes and rotate as needed.

Workday Default

- **Wake:** Open curtains, electrolytes + water, 10-minute walk
- **Breakfast:** Protein + fruit
- **Lunch:** Protein + vegetables + smart carbs
- **Afternoon:** Sunlight exposure + 5-minute breath reset
- **Dinner:** Protein + vegetables; kitchen closed 3 hours before bed
- **Wind-down:** Journal five lines, stretch five minutes, bedtime within your window

Travel Default

- Follow the **Rule of Three:** water, protein, steps
- Pack snacks: jerky, whey, nuts; at airports, order protein + veg
- Walk terminals; light mobility in hotel room

- Maintain peptide timing close to home routine; store per instructions

Weekend Default

- Longer walk or hike; batch-cook proteins and prep vegetables
- Social meals? Anchor with protein; enjoy dessert slowly, once
- Keep bedtime within 60 minutes of weekday schedule, your Monday brain will thank you

Recovery Default

- Contrast shower or sauna if available
- Mobility + Zone-2 walk
- Nap if sleep debt is high; otherwise, protect nighttime window
- Extra collagen scoop and hydration; zero guilt for choosing rest

Why defaults work: They shrink decision fatigue. When life changes, your system doesn't.

The One-Goal Month

Most relapses start with **overreach**: chasing fat loss, muscle, and a marathon all at once. The key is focus, pick **one dominant goal each month** and run the loop.

- **Month A:** Fat Loss → Stack A + 4-week meal plan + step goals
- **Month B:** Muscle → Rebuild Stack + progressive overload + muscle-phase meals
- **Month C:** Skin → Beauty Stack + retinoid cadence + sleep discipline
- **Month D:** Sustain → Minimal signals; consolidate routines

Repeat with small refinements. Over a year, the compounding effect is dramatic, without burnout.

Maintenance Metrics That Matter

Forget chasing arbitrary numbers on a scale. Track signals that predict long-term success. Your 30-Day Journal mirrors these inputs:

- **Sleep Score (1–10):** The master variable for recovery.
- **Morning Energy (1–10):** Honest read on stress versus capacity.

- **Waist (cm or inches):** Composition trend that matters most.
- **Strength Anchor:** Track one push, one pull, and one leg lift (reps or load).
- **Mood Line:** One sentence per night about stress, joy, or mindset.

Five lines a day is enough. When **three of five metrics trend up for two weeks**, maintain course. If not, **adjust sleep and protein** before tinkering with peptide stacks.

Troubleshooting: If This, Do That (7–10 Days)

Challenge	Likely Cause	Quick Fix
Sleep slipping	Late screens / irregular wake time	Screen-off 60 min before bed; same alarm daily; consider DSIP support
Stubborn fat pockets	Stress snacking / high cortisol	Close kitchen 3 hrs pre-bed; +1,500 steps/day; protein at dinner
Flat workouts	Under-recovered muscles	Deload volume by 30%; increase carbs around training; BPC-157 for aches
Joint grumbles	Overuse / low omega-3	Add omega-3s; daily mobility flow
Skin dullness	Low protein / poor sleep	Collagen + vitamin C; earlier lights-out; topical GHK-Cu
Mood dips	Low light / too much caffeine	Morning sunlight; cap caffeine at 2 p.m.; Selank micro-dose AM

Note: *Small, targeted course corrections beat big overhauls. Track your progress in your journal daily for clarity.*

The Travel Playbook: Stay Consistent Anywhere

Pack Your Anchors

- Shaker bottle, whey or collagen packets, jerky, electrolytes.
- Label and store peptides according to stability guidance. Prioritize night-time stacks; skip others if necessary.

Scout Local Essentials

- Find a grocery store within walking distance of your lodging for easy access to protein, veggies, and healthy snacks.

Hotel Routine

- Open curtains immediately upon waking.
- Take hallway or room steps to hit your step goal.
- Bedtime within ±60 minutes of your home window.

Restaurant Strategy

- Base each meal on protein + vegetables.
- Add a starch if you trained that day.

Non-Negotiable

- Walk after your largest meal, digestion, sleep, and waistline will thank you.

When to Cycle Again: 3 Questions to Ask

After every **Sustain** phase, check your metrics before starting a new cycle:

1. **Sleep:** Are you getting 7–8 hours most nights?
   - **If no:** Fix sleep first, cycles won't work on exhaustion.
2. **Morning Energy:** Is your baseline ≥ 7/10 most days?
   - **If no:** Deload or maintain until energy stabilizes.
3. **Goal Clarity:** Do you have one clear focus for the next 4–8 weeks?
   - **If yes:** Proceed with your next cycle.

Key Principle: Let your data guide your decisions, not impulse or mood. This prevents overtraining, burnout, or wasted cycles.

The Five Forever Habits: Your 80/20 Essentials

These five habits are the backbone of the Power Lifestyle System. They're simple, measurable, and powerful enough to keep results compounding even when life gets busy.

1 | Sleep Window
Keep bedtime and wake time within ±60 minutes every day.
Stabilizes hormones, recovery, and mood.
2 | Protein Anchor
30–40 g of quality protein per meal + collagen most days.
Supports metabolism, peptide signaling, and satiety.
3 | Daily Steps
8–10 k steps, preferably outdoors.
Reduces inflammation, balances blood sugar, clears mental fog.
4 | Strength Practice
Lift, push, or pull 2–3 times per week, 20 minutes minimum.
Protects muscle, joints, and hormone responsiveness.
5 | Sun + Breath
Morning sunlight within 10 minutes of waking + one 3-minute breath break midday.
Calms the nervous system and resets energy.
Practice these for a month and you'll feel the shift.
In Sustain & Expand (Chapter 13) you'll learn how to **evolve** these habits season-by-season so they keep growing with you.

Mindset Upgrade: From Motivation to Identity

Motivation vs. Identity

- **Motivation:** loud, pushes, fades.
- **Identity:** quiet, steady, acts automatically.

Shift Your Language:

- Stop saying: "I'm trying to be healthy."
- Start saying: "I'm the kind of person who honors my word."

Result:

- Habits become proof, not punishment.
- Workouts, walks, early bedtimes = evidence you keep promises to yourself.
- Discipline becomes natural; relapse is rare; recovery from setbacks is fast.

Power Prompt:

1. Pick **one small promise** to keep daily for 30 days.
2. Make it take **under 10 minutes**.
3. Track it. Protect it.
4. Watch how it quietly reshapes your self-identity.

Key Takeaway:
The goal isn't doing more. It's becoming the person who always follows through.

Real-World Stories: Momentum That Sticks

Theo, 45: The Consistency Threshold

- He stopped toggling between bulks and cuts. Instead, he ran the Stabilize → Build (fat loss) → Peak → Deload → Sustain loop, then repeated it with a muscle-focus goal. Twelve months later, his waist dropped four inches at the same body weight, true recomposition, not just weight loss.

Amara, 54: Sleep First, Always

- She prioritized a disciplined wind-down routine. Only after sleep averaged 8/10 did she layer in a fat-loss signal. The result? Effortless progress: her clothes fit differently first, then the scale reflected the change.

Gabe, 39: Travel Without Backsliding

- He adopted the Travel Default, keeping only his night-time stack. The secret wasn't the hotel gym, it was post-dinner walks and protein breakfasts. He returned from trips lighter, not heavier, and maintained momentum seamlessly.

The Power Wellness Playbook

When life gets chaotic, return to this blueprint. Think of it as your reset switch, one clear, repeatable system designed to bring energy, recovery, and focus back into balance.

Goal

Focus on one target at a time.

- Whether it's fat loss, energy, recovery, or longevity, clarity drives progress.
- Scatter focus, and everything slows.

Stack

- Use two or three peptide signals at most. Precision beats overload.
- Choose peptides that complement each other, not compete, and allow your body time to adapt before adding more.

Food

Prioritize protein at every meal.

- Time carbs around movement to fuel training and recovery.
- Keep the rest of your plate clean, colorful, and simple.

Sleep

Protect your sleep window as non-negotiable.

- Consistency, not just hours, resets hormones, growth signals, and energy.

Movement

Base your week on strength + steps.

- 2–3 strength sessions preserve muscle.
- Daily walking keeps metabolism and mood steady.

Review

End each week with a quick Journal scan.

- Note what worked, what drained you, and what needs adjusting.
- Your data is your feedback loop, use it to refine, not judge.

Cycle

Stabilize → Build → Peak → Deload → Sustain → Repeat.

- This rhythm **protects results** and prevents burnout.
- When life feels off, you're likely **between phases**, reset and re-sync.

This isn't a plan, it's a **compass**.

Use it anytime you drift, and it will guide you back to **progress**, balance, and momentum that lasts

Frequently Asked Questions

Will I lose progress during deloads?

No. Deloads lock in gains and prevent plateaus. Recovery is progress.

Can I mix goal stacks?

Not at first. Run one primary goal for 4–8 weeks. Layer only when sleep and energy are consistently high.

What if I miss a dose or a workout?
Just pick up where you left off. Rhythm beats perfection.

How long should I stay in Sustain?
As long as you feel great. Many hold it for months, it's your body's steady state of success.

What's the minimum effective plan?

- Consistent sleep window
- Protein at each meal
- 7–8k steps daily
- 2 strength sessions weekly
- One night-time stack

Simplicity scales. This foundation keeps your progress alive, even on your busiest weeks.

Your Closing Charge

You don't need hacks or heroics. You need a repeatable system, one that respects biology and fits real life.

The Power Lifestyle System gives you exactly that: a clear loop that protects your wins and multiplies them.

Run the loop. Trust your Journal. Adjust with data.

And when people ask what changed, tell them the truth: "I stopped fighting my body. I started speaking its language."

By now, you understand how peptides communicate with your cells, how nutrition and movement amplify those signals, and how rhythm, not perfection, creates lasting progress. Now it's time to cover what matters most before you take another step: safety. Peptides are powerful tools, but power only works when paired with respect.

This next chapter gives you a clear framework to:

- Source peptides from trusted, verified suppliers
- Store and handle them properly
- Stack intelligently and dose responsibly
- Know when to pause, reset, or simplify

Because longevity isn't about doing more, it's about doing what works, safely, for the long haul. Smart stacking protects your **results**, your **wallet**, and your **health**, all at once.

CHAPTER 11

SAFETY, SOURCING & STACKING THE SMART WAY

Every meaningful transformation begins with respect for the process. Peptides are not shortcuts or magic fixes; they are communication tools that work best when paired with awareness, discipline, and consistency. When you understand what each compound does, how it interacts with your system, and when to step back, you move from trial and error to true mastery. Safety is not about restriction; it is about creating stability so your body can do what it's designed to do: heal, grow, and thrive. The goal is not to rush results but to build a foundation strong enough to sustain them.

Key Principles for Safe and Effective Peptide Use:

- **Precision:** Know what you are taking, why you are taking it, and how it fits into your larger plan.
- **Patience:** Allow time for adaptation. Your body changes in rhythms, not in shortcuts.
- **Integrity:** Follow verified protocols and source responsibly from trusted suppliers.
- **Consistency:** Regularly tracking sleep, energy, and recovery provides data-driven insights, not guesswork.
- **Self-Awareness:** Tune into how your body responds. Small signs often reveal what needs adjusting.

Safety is not a limitation; it is your greatest advantage. By approaching peptides with respect and intention, you create the conditions for lasting transformation, progress that feels steady, sustainable, and entirely within your control.

The Power Wellness Promise

Peptides are not shortcuts; they're intelligent biological messengers designed to help your body repair, rebuild, and perform at its best. When used with care and respect, they amplify what's already possible within you. But when approached carelessly, they lose their potential and may even invite unnecessary risk. True mastery comes from treating peptides as precision tools, not experiments. Your results depend as much on your methods as on the molecules themselves.

The Three Pillars of Safe Progress:

- **Purity:** Use only verified, pharmaceutical-grade ingredients from trusted and transparent sources.
- **Precision:** Follow accurate dosing, maintain sterile technique, and document every cycle in your Journal.
- **Patience:** Respect natural timelines. Allow full recovery and receptor resets between cycles.

Safety isn't a restriction; it's the foundation that makes every result sustainable. The more disciplined your process, the more dependable your outcomes. Think of safety as part of the system itself: when it's built into your rhythm, progress feels effortless and lasting.

Disclaimer: *Always consult a qualified healthcare professional before starting or adjusting any peptide protocol. Safe progress begins with expert guidance and informed choices.*

Spotting Legitimate Sources

In a growing market filled with promises, knowing how to separate trustworthy peptide suppliers from risky ones protects both your results and your health. Peptides are precision compounds, not casual supplements, so sourcing from credible providers is your first safety checkpoint. A legitimate supplier operates transparently, documents quality, and maintains pharmaceutical-level standards throughout the production and packaging process. If any part of that chain feels vague or exaggerated, that's your cue to pause and verify before you buy.

What to Look For

- **GMP Certification:** "Good Manufacturing Practice" verified facility ensures pharmaceutical-grade production.
- **Third-Party COA (Certificate of Analysis):** Includes batch number and at least **98% purity**.
- **Sterile Vials & Seals:** Clear powder with no residue, cracks, or discoloration.
- **Transparent Labeling:** Must list peptide name, lot number, quantity (mg), and expiration date.

Avoid These

- Colored, cloudy, or clumpy powder.
- "Pre-mixed super stacks" or blends without precise dosages.
- Sellers without a valid COA or those using vague "lab-tested" claims.
- Marketing that guarantees instant or dramatic results.

PRO TIP

Reputable longevity clinics and licensed compounding pharmacies can quickly verify authenticity, far more reliably than unregulated "research" sites online.

"For Research Use Only": What It Really Means

Seeing "For Research Use Only" on a peptide label can feel confusing, but it's not a red flag by itself. This phrase doesn't mean the peptide is illegal; it simply indicates that it hasn't been approved for over-the-counter sale or general consumer distribution.

Clinics, under licensed medical supervision, can legally **prescribe and compound** these same peptides for therapeutic use. The label is primarily a **regulatory safeguard**, ensuring that only qualified professionals or educated users handle these compounds responsibly.

If you're studying peptides independently, this label serves as a clear reminder:

- You are responsible for **sterile preparation and accurate dosing.**
- You must track **responses and side effects** with honesty and precision.
- You are working with **bioactive molecules**, not casual supplements.

Think of *"research use only"* as a boundary line, one that separates curiosity from carelessness, and responsibility from risk.

Reconstitution & Storage Essentials

Peptides are delicate molecules that arrive as a **freeze-dried (lyophilized) powder** to preserve stability during shipping. To activate them safely and maintain potency, you'll need to reconstitute and store them with precision. Think of this as chemistry in the service of consistency, every step helps ensure your results come from purity, not chance.

You'll Need:

- Bacteriostatic water (0.9% benzyl alcohol)
- Alcohol swabs
- 1 mL insulin syringes (100 units)

Safe Mixing Method:

1. Wipe vial tops thoroughly with alcohol to prevent contamination.
2. Draw bacteriostatic water **slowly**, allowing it to slide down the vial wall, **never spray directly** onto the powder.
3. Swirl the vial gently until the solution clears, **do not shake.**
4. Label the vial with the **date mixed** for easy tracking.

Storage Guidelines:

- Store refrigerated between **36°F and 46°F (2 °C–8°C).**
- Discard after **30 days** or sooner if the solution becomes **cloudy or discolored.**

These small details, sterility, temperature, and timing, are what separate safe, effective use from wasted potential. Handle peptides like precision tools, and they'll reward you with reliable, lasting performance.

Educational Example: Reconstituting BPC-157 (5 mg Vial)

(For Informational and Educational Purposes Only)

Understanding the math and method behind reconstitution helps you visualize proper dosing and sterile handling. This example demonstrates a typical setup using **BPC-157 (5 mg vial)** to illustrate how concentration and measurement align.

Each vial contains: 5 mg (5,000 mcg) of peptide

Step-by-Step Reconstitution:

1. Using a sterile syringe, add **2 mL of bacteriostatic water** slowly down the side of the vial.
2. **Swirl gently** until the powder fully dissolves (do not shake).

Your solution now equals **2,500 mcg per mL.**
That means **every 0.1 mL (10 syringe units) ≈ 250 mcg of BPC-157.**

Example Calculation:

Step	Result
250 mcg ÷ 2,500 mcg/mL	= 0.10 mL
0.10 mL × 100 units/mL	= 10 syringe units

Draw 10 units (0.10 mL) ≈ 250 mcg.
Quick Reference (5 mg + 2 mL BAC Water):

Desired Amount	mL to Draw	Syringe Mark
100 mcg	0.04 mL	4 units
250 mcg	0.10 mL	10 units
500 mcg	0.20 mL	20 units
750 mcg	0.30 mL	30 units
1,000 mcg (1 mg)	0.40 mL	40 units

Label Example:
BPC-157 5 mg / 2 mL = 2,500 mcg per mL
Storage:
Refrigerate between **36–46°F (2–8°C)** and **discard after 30 days** or if the solution becomes cloudy.

Disclaimer: *This example is for* ***educational purposes only*** *to illustrate calculation principles and safe handling concepts. It is* ***not medical advice*** *or a treatment guide. Always consult a qualified healthcare professional for personalized evaluation before using any peptide or injectable compound.*

Precision & Injection Technique

Proper technique ensures safety, reduces irritation, and protects tissue integrity. Repeated injections in the same spot without rotation can lead to bruising, lumps, or the formation of scar tissue.

Rotation Keeps Tissue Healthy

- Common sites: **abdomen** (2 inches from navel), **front of thigh**, **back of triceps**
- Rotate sites in sequence: **right abdomen → left abdomen → right thigh → left thigh → repeat**

Technique Snapshot

1. **Clean** the injection site with an alcohol swab
2. **Pinch** a ½-inch skin fold to lift subcutaneous tissue
3. **Insert** the needle at **45–90°** depending on depth and syringe type
4. **Inject slowly** and withdraw gently to minimize tissue trauma
5. **Apply light pressure** with a swab, do not massage the area

Watch for adverse signs:

- Redness larger than 2 inches
- Persistent pain or swelling

If either occurs, **pause injections** and assess the situation before continuing.

Consistent rotation and careful technique ensure injections remain effective, comfortable, and safe, supporting optimal peptide absorption and minimizing complications.

When to Pause, Cycle, or Switch

Even the most effective peptide stacks benefit from structured breaks. These pauses allow your body to reset receptors, support hormone balance, and prevent diminishing returns.

Typical Stack Rhythm

- **Growth-hormone or repair peptides**: 8–12 weeks active → 4 weeks off
- **Immune or sleep stacks**: 2–4 weeks active → 1–2 weeks off

Signals to Pause Immediately

- Sleep consistently drops below 6 hours for three nights
- Resting heart rate rises more than 10 bpm above your normal baseline
- New rash, persistent bloating, or unusual digestive issues appear
- Significant mood swings or energy crashes

Practical Guidance

- Always **track changes in your Journal** to identify patterns early
- Consult a qualified clinician before resuming or switching stacks
- Treat these pause points as part of the system, not failures; listening to your body preserves safety and maximizes long-term results

Following a thoughtful cycle and pause strategy ensures you maintain the benefits of peptides while minimizing risk and supporting sustainable wellness.

Legal & Ethical Clarity

Peptides are primarily classified as research biologics by the FDA. They may be legally compounded under a licensed prescription or used in sanctioned clinical research. Claims in retail marketing suggesting that peptides "cure," "treat," or produce instant fat loss are not allowed. Understanding this distinction helps protect your safety and keeps your approach compliant.

Ethical Peptide Use Guidelines

- Never double-dose in an attempt to speed results
- Do not share vials or supplies with others
- Dispose of needles and syringes in approved sharps containers
- Maintain accurate purchase and usage records for traceability
- Treat each protocol with integrity to safeguard both your health and the credibility of the wellness community

Respecting legal boundaries and ethical standards ensures that your peptide use is both safe and responsible. Following these guidelines helps preserve your results, your well-being, and the trustworthiness of the biohacking and wellness community.

Power Wellness Safety Checklist

Keep this checklist visible near your mixing and injection area to ensure consistent safety and precision:

- Wash your hands thoroughly and wipe all surfaces before handling peptides.
- Use only bacteriostatic water for reconstitution.
- Clearly label each vial with the mixing date and intended dose.
- Store vials upright in the refrigerator (36–46 °F / 2–8 °C).
- Rotate injection sites daily to protect tissue health.
- Discard any vial after 30 days or if the solution becomes cloudy or discolored.
- Record every dose, time, and site in your Journal for accurate tracking.
- Never inject if the solution appears cloudy, colored, or shows particles.

Following this checklist consistently ensures potency, reduces the risk of infection or irritation, and keeps your peptide program both safe and effective over time.

Final Note

Safety isn't a restriction, it's a strategy. The more precise you are with sourcing, mixing, and tracking, the faster and safer your results will come. Every protocol becomes more effective when it's built on discipline and respect for the process.

Clarity creates confidence. Confidence sustains consistency. Consistency builds transformation. Respect the signal. Track the response. Own the results. The smarter you practice, the longer your progress lasts.

You've built the foundation: clear signals, safe stacks, strong habits. Now it's time to put it all into motion. The **30-Day Power Reset** is your step-by-step system to synchronize peptides, nutrition, and movement into one focused rhythm. This isn't a challenge or a cleanse, it's a reset. It's a guided month designed to realign energy, metabolism, and recovery so your results compound automatically.

This blueprint walks you through daily structure, weekly focus, and simple metrics to track real progress: fat loss, energy, sleep quality, and mental clarity. In just four weeks, you'll see that transformation doesn't require chaos, only consistency with direction.

You've learned the science. Now it's time to live the system.

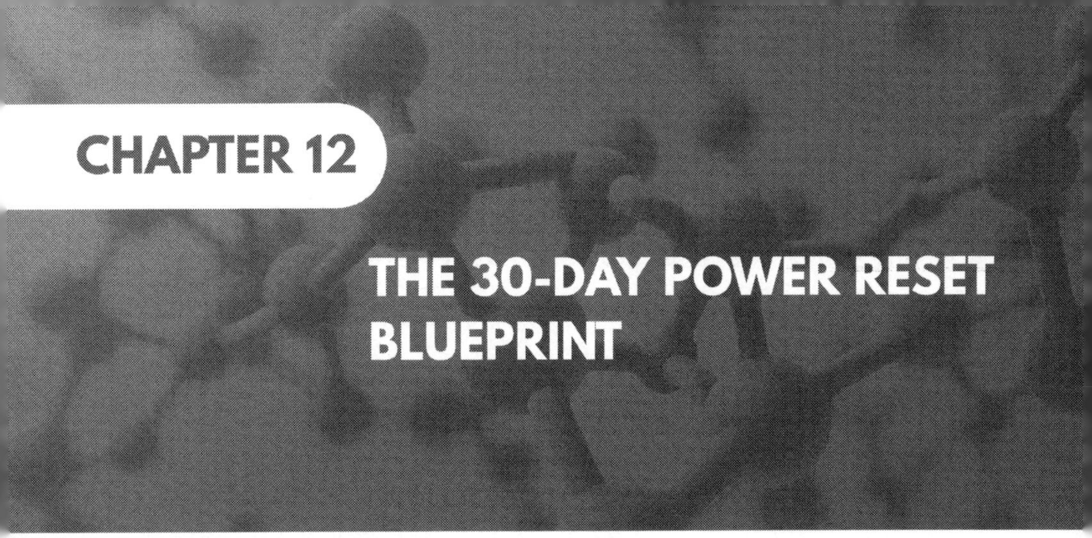

CHAPTER 12

THE 30-DAY POWER RESET BLUEPRINT

Your Fast-Track Plan to Feel and See Results: Starting Now

Most health programs end with more information. This one ends with transformation. The Power Reset Blueprint removes the guesswork: no complicated schedules, no confusion about timing, no overwhelm about what to do next. It's a clear, step-by-step guide that shows you exactly how to align your peptides, nutrition, movement, and mindset for maximum impact.

Think of this as your 30-day accelerator, a focused reset that reconnects your metabolism, hormones, and recovery rhythm. In just four weeks, your body will remember how to communicate efficiently again: better sleep, steadier energy, improved digestion, and visible changes in your physique.

Each day builds on the last with simple, repeatable actions that deliver compounding results. You won't chase motivation, you'll build momentum through rhythm and structure. By the end, you'll understand how to maintain progress without burnout or restriction.

This isn't another plan to follow; it's a system designed to make progress automatic. The blueprint helps you work with your biology, not against it, so you can move, rest, and recover with confidence.
Your body already knows how to thrive. This 30-day reset simply teaches it to listen again.

How the Blueprint Works

The Power Reset Blueprint runs on the same Power Lifestyle Loop you've already mastered: **Stabilize → Build → Peak → Deload.**
Each phase lasts just long enough to create adaptation, without overwhelm or burnout.

Every day follows four simple checkpoints designed to anchor your progress and make results automatic:

1. Power Pillar: Focus

Start with clarity. Choose one peptide goal and apply the matching stack, fat loss, recovery, or beauty. Precision replaces randomness.

2. Support: Nourish & Hydrate

Eat and drink on rhythm using your Power Meal Plan. Each meal becomes a message to your metabolism: "You're safe, fueled, and ready to rebuild."

3. Stack: Move & Recover

Train or restore intentionally. Rotate between strength, steps, and mobility so energy stays high and inflammation stays low.

4. Sustain: Reflect & Reset

End your day with five simple lines: sleep score, energy, mood, gratitude, and tomorrow's intention. Reflection keeps the loop alive.

That's it, four deliberate moves per day that keep you progressing without confusion. Simple enough to repeat. Powerful enough to transform.

Week 1: Stabilize: Reset Your Rhythm

This first week is all about rebalancing your internal clock and restoring the foundation of health: calm digestion, stable energy, and quality sleep. Before you chase performance or physique goals, your system must first feel safe and predictable. Stability isn't slow, it's the launchpad for everything that follows.

Goal: calm inflammation, balance energy, and restore deep, consistent sleep.
Focus: routine, recovery, and rhythm.

Daily Targets

- Wake and sleep within a 60-minute window.
- Get morning light exposure followed by a 10-minute walk.
- Eat protein at every meal (about 30 g minimum).
- Hydrate with at least half your body weight (in ounces) of water daily.
- Add one 20-minute zone-2 walk after dinner.

Stack Example: baseline support only, use a gentle sleep or gut stack if needed.

Expected Result: calmer digestion, less bloating, and steady morning energy.

Power Tip: *Don't chase fat loss yet, chase rhythm. When your sleep, hydration, and meals run on schedule, your metabolism follows.* Consistency this week sets the stage for acceleration next week.

Week 2: Build: Activate Change

With your rhythm now steady, it's time to build momentum. Week 2 shifts from stabilization to activation, where nutrition, movement, and recovery begin working in sync. The focus is simple: feed your body well, move with purpose, and maintain the consistency you earned last week. This is where your metabolism starts to trust the process.

Goal: increase nutrient density and introduce structured movement.

Focus: muscle tone, digestion, and nutrient delivery.

Daily Targets

- Complete two resistance-training sessions this week and hit 8,000 steps per day.
- Add colorful fruits and vegetables to every meal to boost micronutrient intake.
- Include omega-3 fats from sources like salmon, chia, or flax for joint and brain support.
- Keep your bedtime consistent and power down screens at least one hour before sleep.
- Use collagen or electrolytes as needed to aid muscle recovery and hydration.

Stack Example: maintain your base peptide; optionally add collagen or a repair signal (such as BPC-157).

Expected Result: elevated energy, firmer muscle tone, and stronger appetite control.

Power Tip: *Think quality over quantity, your recovery determines how much you can grow.*

Week 3: Peak: Precision and Consistency

You've built the foundation, now it's time to sharpen your edge. Week 3 is about refinement and precision, where small details separate effort from excellence. This phase isn't about doing *more*; it's about doing what works, consistently and cleanly. Every meal, workout, and recovery choice now compounds your progress.

Goal: refine execution and harvest visible results.
Focus: protein timing, training intensity, and stress control.
Daily Targets

- Complete three strength or interval sessions this week, train with intention, not exhaustion.
- Commit to 100% adherence to your meal plan; minimize or eliminate alcohol and added sugars.
- Journal nightly to identify your **Best-Day Pattern**, the habits, timing, and mindset that make you feel your best.
- Sleep at least seven hours and cut caffeine by 2 p.m. to preserve recovery quality.

Stack Example: maintain your primary goal stack (fat loss, skin, or muscle).
Add only **one** supportive peptide if your energy has averaged 8/10 or higher for two consecutive weeks.
Expected Result: sharper focus, deeper sleep, and clear physical changes, your rhythm is paying off.

Power Tip: *Protect your recovery like a workout, your results depend on it.*

Week 4: Deload & Reflect

This is the reset before the next rise. Week 4 is where recovery becomes strategy, not rest for rest's sake, but intentional recalibration. You're not losing progress; you're locking it in. By allowing receptors, hormones, and your nervous system to reset, you ensure that every future cycle begins from strength, not fatigue.

Goal: consolidate gains, reset receptors, and prepare for your next cycle.
Focus: recovery and reflection.
Daily Targets

- Two mobility or yoga sessions to restore flexibility and joint integrity.
- Daily 30-minute walk outdoors to keep circulation and mood steady.
- Extend sleep to 8 hours per night, your body upgrades itself while you rest.
- Return to maintenance calories with protein-rich meals.
- Reflect on which habits felt natural and easy to sustain.

Stack Example: pause goal-specific peptides; continue only sleep or repair support.
Expected Result: a refreshed nervous system, stable mood, and renewed motivation.

Power Prompt: *"What felt effortless this week?"*
Your next cycle should feel exactly like that, smooth, aligned, and sustainable.

Quick-View Daily Template

Time	Focus	Example
Morning	Water + light + protein	16 oz water, eggs + berries, 10-min walk
Midday	Movement + hydration	30-min lift or walk, electrolytes
Evening	Stack + screens-off hour	Inject (if applicable), stretch 5 min
Journal	5 lines	Energy / Sleep / Mood / Gratitude / Plan

The goal isn't perfection, it's rhythm. These anchors turn small daily wins into long-term transformation.

Tracking the Five Core Metrics

Metric	Target	Why It Matters
Sleep (hours)	7+	Recovery = repair
Energy (score)	1–10	Feedback on recovery
Waist (inches/cm)	—	Composition trend
Steps	8,000–10,000	Metabolic stability
Mood line	😁 🙂 😐 ☹️ 😫	Mind–body connection

Progress Rule:
When **three of five metrics improve by more than 20%**, you're ready to move into your next **Build** or **Sustain** phase.

Power Reset Checklist

- **Pick one goal:** fat loss · muscle · joint · skin
- **Choose your matching stack card** from the Toolkit
- **Follow the four-phase rhythm:** Stabilize → Build → Peak → Deload
- **Use your Journal and Meal Plan** for daily accountability
- **Re-evaluate your metrics** on Day 30

Simple = Sustainable.
Consistency, not complexity, creates change.

Example in Motion

Ethan, 41: "From Stuck to Steady."
Ethan started with a simple plan: nightly **CJC-1295 + Ipamorelin**, **protein-first meals**, and **8,000 steps a day**.
By **Day 10**, his sleep extended by 45 minutes.
By **Day 28**, his waist measured **1.5 inches smaller**.

His reflection captures the Power Reset effect: "I finally know what to do each day, no guessing, no overwhelm."

That clarity not intensity is what makes transformation sustainable.

Transition Next

At **Day 30**, you'll know your baseline of what foods, stacks, and routines give you calm, sustained energy. From here, you can either start another **Build → Peak → Deload** loop or move into the **Sustain Phase** outlined in the next chapter.

Momentum is medicine. Structure creates freedom. Thirty days from now, you'll see that power isn't something you find it's something you repeat.

You've proven what your body can do in just thirty days. Now it's time to make those results **effortless**. Transformation isn't the finish line, it's the foundation. True power begins when your new habits no longer feel like effort but identity. You don't have to start over because these practices have become who you are.

This chapter will teach you how to **stabilize progress, prevent backslides, and keep growing** without burnout or obsession. You'll learn to read your body's signals, cycle intelligently, and expand results across **strength, focus, skin, and longevity**. Real success isn't built on intensity, it's built on **stability that compounds**.

You've reset the system. Now it's time to live in balance, **strong, steady, and self-powered for life**.

CHAPTER 13

SUSTAIN & EXPAND: HOW TO KEEP RESULTS FOR LIFE

Over the past 30 days, you've done more than just follow a program, you've awakened your body's innate intelligence. Each meal, movement, and mindful choice has strengthened your system and fine-tuned the signals that keep you energized, balanced, and resilient. What might have felt like small, daily actions were actually rewiring your body from the inside out. You've proven to yourself that your body is not fragile; it is adaptable, responsive, and capable of cellular-level recovery. Now, instead of constantly pushing for transformation, the focus shifts toward preserving the progress you've made. This isn't about extreme regimens or endless experimentation. It's about understanding what works for you, maintaining consistency, and nurturing your body to stay strong, youthful, and vibrant for the long term. By leaning into these tools and practices, you'll continue to support your body's natural rhythm, protect your energy, and ensure that the gains you've worked for become effortless and lasting.

Key Points

- Your body is responsive, not fragile, and has proven its ability to adapt.
- The past 30 days have strengthened your cellular systems and improved internal communication.
- Consistency in movement, nutrition, and recovery has created lasting internal renewal.
- The focus now shifts from transformation to preservation and maintenance.

- Tools and practices exist to help you stay strong, resilient, and youthful without requiring constant resets.
- Sustaining results is easier when you understand and respect your body's signals.
- Actual vitality comes from long-term habits, not short-term extremes.

Preservation is the next step in your journey. With the foundation you've built, maintaining strength, energy, and balance becomes second nature. This chapter equips you with the guidance to keep your body resilient and youthful, ensuring that every choice reinforces the gains you've earned. Your progress is not temporary, it is a lasting reflection of your commitment and your body's incredible ability to respond and thrive.

From Reset to Rhythm

Every reset ignites a spark, but lasting health isn't about one-time effort, it's about rhythm. True wellness comes from **patterns that repeat so often they become effortless**, moving from conscious effort to instinctive action. Early on, you tracked sleep, meals, and peptide stacks to stay aware. That awareness was essential, but the next step is automaticity: doing what works without relying on motivation or willpower.

The formula is simple: Awareness → Consistency → Identity. Each habit progresses from a checklist to an instinct, eventually becoming ingrained in your biology. Over time, the system you built replaces the plan. You're no longer "following a regimen", you're living a structure that works, day in and day out, without friction.

When rhythm takes over, results compound naturally. Energy stabilizes, digestion smooths, workouts feel easier, and your habits stop requiring thought, they **become who you are**. The spark of reset evolves into a steady flame of identity, lighting the way for every next level of health, performance, and vitality.

Living in the Sustain Phase

The Sustain Phase is where your progress becomes durable and effortless. Unlike other phases, you're not chasing rapid change, you're **protecting and refining** the results you've built. Think of Sustain not in weeks, but in seasons. Each quarter of the year has a focus that keeps your body balanced, resilient, and primed for the next cycle when you choose to begin again.

Seasonal Focus & Adjustments:

- **Winter – Recovery & Hormone Balance**
- Prioritize rest, warmth, grounding foods, and gentle movement. Let your nervous system recover fully.
- **Spring – Gut & Detox Renewal**
- Introduce fresh greens, probiotics, and lighter, more dynamic movement. Support digestion and energy.
- **Summer – Energy & Physique**
- Train outdoors, hydrate deeply, and temporarily deload goal-specific peptides. Celebrate your performance and vitality.
- **Autumn – Immunity & Repair**
- Emphasize omega-3s, vitamin D, sauna or cold therapy, and supportive recovery practices. Prepare your system for winter.

In Sustain, you're not restarting cycles, you're **evolving through them**. By aligning your lifestyle, nutrition, movement, and recovery with seasonal rhythms, your body stays in harmony, results compound naturally, and wellness becomes an integral part of your identity rather than an effort.

Peptide Maintenance & Cycling

Once you've established a strong foundation, consistent sleep, nutrition, and movement, peptides are no longer daily necessities. They become **precision tools** that support targeted goals when used thoughtfully. Cycles, not constant use, allow your body to respond effectively without overstimulation or dependency.

Typical Peptide Cycles by Goal:

- **Fat Management**

    - **Frequency:** 1–2 cycles per year
    - **Example Signals:** CJC-1295 + Ipamorelin, 8–12 weeks
- **Joint Recovery**
    - **Frequency:** As needed
    - **Example Signals:** BPC-157 microdose 2–3 times per week
- **Skin & Sleep**
    - **Frequency:** Quarterly reset
    - **Example Signals:** GHK-Cu or Epitalon, 10–14 days
- **Immune or Gut Support**
    - **Frequency:** Seasonal
    - **Example Signals:** TA-1 or KPV rotation

The goal of cycling is **precision, not dependence**. Your body already knows how to repair, regulate, and maintain itself. Peptides simply **remind your cells of their natural capabilities**, amplifying results while keeping your system resilient. Using them in rhythm ensures that every cycle contributes to long-term health, efficiency, and effortless maintenance.

Data That Defines Longevity

Longevity isn't measured by weight or trends on a scale, it's revealed in **functional markers that show how well your body actually works**. By focusing on the signals your body gives you, you can assess youthfulness, recovery, and metabolic resilience without the need for expensive tests. Tracking the correct data enables you to **intervene early, optimize routines, and maintain your vitality**.

Five Key Longevity Markers:

- **Sleep Score**: quality recovery equals cellular repair and hormonal balance.
- **Grip Strength / Push-Up Test**: muscular strength predicts lifespan and functional independence.
- **Waist Circumference**: a reliable measure of metabolic health and visceral fat.
- **Mood & Focus Quality:** balanced neurochemistry supports resilience, clarity, and stress adaptation.
- **Inflammation Index**: low systemic inflammation signals a quietly running, efficient body.

Consistently monitoring these five metrics gives you actionable insight into your biological age.

The Expansion Mindset

Sustainability isn't just about maintaining stability; it's about **amplifying your impact and influence**. Once you've mastered your personal health loop, the same principles that optimized your body can optimize every area of life. Expansion means **leveraging your consistency and clarity** to grow outcomes, relationships, and resilience without extra stress or effort.

Ways to Expand Your Power:

- **Teach What You Know**: Share your routines, habits, and insights with friends, family, or workout partners. Teaching reinforces mastery and creates accountability.
- **Apply the Loop to New Domains**: Use Signal → Support → Stack → Sustain for your career, creative projects, or personal relationships. Systems that work for biology work for life.
- **Set New PRs for Peace**: Track progress not only in physical goals but in calmer mornings, stronger boundaries, or more focused energy.
- **Lead Through Health**: Your stability, energy, and clarity now become a model others can follow. Health transforms into a leadership skill.

Growth isn't only measured in pounds lifted or calories burned, it's measured in influence, focus, and calm mastery. When your habits become an integral part of your identity, they create ripple effects: **your life, your community, and your performance all benefit**. Expansion begins when sustaining yourself becomes effortless.

Expansion Mindset

You've already proven that rhythm beats motivation. Now, expansion means applying that rhythm beyond health, into focus, relationships, and purpose.

Use the same four-part formula everywhere: **Signal → Support → Stack → Sustain.**

What works for biology works for life.

Growth now feels lighter, not harder.
You're not chasing transformation; you're refining mastery.

Power Wellness Habits for Life

The habits that created your initial results are not just short-term tools, they are **lifelong anchors for health, energy, and resilience**. Once your peptide cycles and structured routines have taught your body what it can do, these five behaviors ensure your system keeps communicating clearly, your energy stays steady, and your progress compounds naturally over time. In Chapter 10, you built your foundation with the Five Forever Habits.

Here's how to *expand* them for lifelong longevity and resilience:

1 | Sleep Window → Sleep Mastery
Protect it across travel and stress seasons. Use light exposure and wind-down rituals to lock circadian rhythm.

2 | Protein Anchor → Metabolic Variety
Keep protein high but rotate sources. Add diverse plants to feed your microbiome and sustain metabolism.

3 | Steps + Strength → Play + Performance
Blend structure with enjoyment—hiking, cycling, yoga, resistance. Movement becomes recreation, not obligation.

4 | Sun + Breath → Stress Regulation
Use morning light to anchor energy and 3-minute breath resets during workdays to calm cortisol.

5 | Reflect & Record → Quarterly Compass
You no longer need daily logs; instead, review monthly or quarterly patterns. Notice trends and course-correct early.

These refined habits keep your biology tuned without effort.
They're not a checklist anymore, they're your operating rhythm.

Longevity Expansion: Beyond Peptides

Once your body's signaling pathways are running smoothly, you've created a foundation for lasting vitality. At this stage, wellness becomes about enhancement, resilience, and compounding benefits, not repair. The strategies you add now should amplify what already works, layering advanced support without replacing the core habits and rhythms that built your results.

Advanced Tools for Longevity:

- **Mitochondrial Peptides**: Compounds like MOTS-c or SS-31, help renew cellular energy and optimize metabolic efficiency.
- **Autophagy Activators**: Use strategic fasting, quality sleep, and zone-2 cardio to stimulate cellular recycling and repair.
- **Microbiome Optimization**: Support gut health with diverse plants, prebiotics, and probiotics, explored in depth in the Gut Fix Power framework.

At this stage, you're no longer just repairing damage, you're **enhancing function, boosting resilience, and future-proofing your biology**. Every new tool should integrate seamlessly with your existing Power Wellness system, ensuring results compound naturally. You've moved from maintaining health to **unlocking the next level of performance and longevity**.

Community & Accountability

Sustainable wellness isn't just a personal journey, it's a social one. Your habits, routines, and progress **thrive when supported and mirrored by others**. Long-term success comes not from fleeting motivation but from consistent action, and accountability makes consistency far easier to maintain.

Ways to Build Support:

- **Accountability Partner** - Check in weekly with someone who tracks habits and progress alongside you.
- **Create a Power Circle** - Form a small network of friends or colleagues committed to sustainable health routines.
- **Collective Momentum** - Group energy and shared goals help you stay consistent when life gets hectic.

Consistency compounds best when it's shared. Accountability doesn't just keep you honest, it multiplies your results. By embedding social support into your Power Wellness system, you protect your rhythm, reinforce habits, and turn individual effort into collective progress. Ultimately, wellness is easier, more enjoyable, and more lasting when it's part of a community that moves forward together.

The Power Wellness Compass

Wellness isn't about constant action, it's about clarity, awareness, and course correction. The Power Wellness Compass provides a simple framework to **check in with your body, habits, and results** on a monthly or quarterly basis. By asking the right questions, you stay aligned with your goals and avoid wasted effort.

Monthly/Quarterly Check-In:

- **What signal is my body sending clearly right now?** → Build **awareness** of energy, recovery, mood, or other core metrics.
- **What stack or habit supports that signal best?** → Ensure **precision** in nutrition, movement, or peptides.
- **Where do I feel friction or resistance?** → Identify areas for **course correction** before small issues become setbacks.
- **What felt effortless this month?** → **Reinforce** habits that naturally stick without forcing willpower.
- **What's one area I can expand next?** → Choose a single focus for **growth** and compounding results.

The process is simple: **Ask → Adjust → Act.** When repeated regularly, this framework transforms occasional progress into predictable, sustainable results. The Power Wellness Compass keeps your health intentional, guided by feedback from your own body, and your actions aligned with what truly matters.

Legacy of Power

True wellness isn't about chasing aesthetics, it's about mastery and control. Over time, you've learned to **hear your body's whispers before they become shouts**, to recognize what supports recovery, energy, and resilience. Confidence now comes from **understanding your biology**, rather than relying on trends or shortcuts.

Core Takeaways:

- **Interpret Signals:** You can sense fatigue, stress, or imbalance early and act before they escalate.
- **Build Confidence:** Your results come from consistency and rhythm, not guesswork.
- **Speak Your Body's Language:** Repair, renewal, and energy are guided by clear communication, nutrition, movement, rest, and optional support signals.
- **Forge Power Through Repetition:** True strength emerges when healthy patterns become automatic and identity-driven.
- **Trust the System:** Follow the loop: Stabilize → Build → Peak → Deload → Sustain and let your body adapt naturally.

Final Reflection

Mastery isn't found in a finish line, it's found in the daily practice of listening, responding, and aligning with your biology. Sustain is not the end; it's the phase where habits, signals, and rhythm become instinct. Over time, you've learned that results come from **precision, patience, and consistency**, not force or extremes.

Key Principles:

- **Communicate, Don't Force:** Your body responds to clear instructions, not pressure.
- **Consistency Over Heroics:** Small, repeated actions compound into lasting transformation.
- **Age as Collaboration:** Longevity and vitality improve when you respect natural rhythms and recovery cycles.
- **Feedback Is Power:** Sleep, energy, mood, and performance are your daily compass.
- **Identity Drives Action:** When health becomes part of who you are, you no longer need motivation to maintain it.

Your body was never broken. It was waiting for better instructions. Now, with knowledge, rhythm, and respect, you know precisely how to give them, and sustain a life of strength, energy, and clarity.

CONCLUSION: Awaken Your Power Wellness

Peptides are not a quick fix. They are a powerful support system that can accelerate your progress when combined with intentional daily practices. They work best when you build a strong foundation of nutrition, recovery, and consistency. Approaching them with the right mindset ensures that you are not just chasing quick results but building lasting health and performance.

Here are the most important points to remember from this guide:

Nutrition comes first. Whole, balanced foods provide the environment peptides need to work effectively. Without this foundation, their impact is limited.

Strategic supplementation matters. Support your body with vitamins, minerals, and other targeted nutrients that enhance rather than compete with peptide protocols.

Recovery is non-negotiable. Quality sleep, hydration, and stress management are just as important as training or supplementation.

Consistency compounds results. Sustainable routines and daily discipline will always outlast short bursts of intensity.

Professional guidance protects you. Legal access and expert oversight ensure safety, purity, and effectiveness of peptides.

Long-term thinking wins. Treat your peptide journey as a lifelong health project rather than a temporary fix.

Peptides open doors to incredible potential, but the real power lies in how you integrate them into a lifestyle of discipline, awareness, and care. By combining science with strategy, you create space for transformation that lasts far beyond the next month or year.

Your journey does not end with the last page of this book. It continues in the daily choices you make; how you eat, how you rest, how you move, and how you stay curious about your own health. When you view peptides not as shortcuts but as partners in your lifelong wellness, you set yourself up to become stronger, sharper, and more resilient with every passing season.

Pause for a moment.
Take a deep breath.
You made it here, not by luck, but by choice.

You picked up this book because something inside you whispered, there has to be more.
More energy.
More clarity.
More life.

You were right. There is more. And it has been inside you all along, waiting for the right signal to wake it up.

Every chapter in this book was written for this moment, standing in the gap for who you were and who you are becoming. You have learned how your body speaks in signals, how your habits translate those signals into chemistry, and how the right strategy can reignite everything you thought you lost.

That is the heart of Power Wellness. It is not another diet, protocol, or promise. It is a reintroduction to the body you were born with, the one that already knows how to repair, rebuild, and thrive when you give it what it needs.

Think about how far you have come while reading these pages. You have learned that fatigue is not weakness; it is feedback. That joint pain is not random; it is your body's way of asking for alignment. That cravings, mood swings, and stubborn fat are not personal failures; they are biochemical messages waiting to be decoded.

And now, you know how to decode them.

When you fuel yourself with clean nutrients, when you sleep deeply, when you recover with intention, and when you move for function rather than punishment, something powerful happens.

Your body starts remembering. Your metabolism resets. Your mind clears. Your motivation ignites.

Small daily actions become momentum. Momentum becomes transformation. Transformation becomes your new normal.

That is not hype; that is biology working for you instead of against you.

Every reader reaches a point where they ask, *Can this really work for me?* The answer is yes, if you keep showing up. Results do not come from perfection; they come from persistence. You have already taken the hardest step: deciding to begin.

From here, your mission is to keep the signal strong. Every choice is a message. Every meal, every night of rest, every moment of gratitude tells your body to keep healing, keep growing, and keep moving forward.

The foundation you have built does not stop here. It compounds. You have learned the framework:

Signal → Support → Stack → Sustain

When you repeat that rhythm, your energy stays elevated, your systems stay balanced, and your results stay real.

That is why Power Wellness is not just a concept; it is a lifestyle designed to make thriving automatic. This is how you defy slow aging, reduce inflammation, and build strength, beauty, and clarity at every age. No gimmicks. No deprivation. Just biology restored to its natural brilliance.

Because the truth is, you do not need to chase youth. You can now communicate with it.

As you close this book, understand that this is not the end. It is the ignition point, the moment you stop surviving and start expanding.

Your body knows what to do. Your mind knows what it wants. Now your only job is to stay consistent.

You have awakened your Power Wellness System.
Protect it. Strengthen it. Share it.

Let your results speak for what is possible. Let your energy inspire others. Because the real revolution does not happen in clinics or labs; it happens in the quiet, daily moments when someone like you decides to live differently.

That is how the movement grows: one signal, one choice, one believer at a time.

You are that believer.
You are that signal.
You are the proof.

So go live it. Powerfully.

REFERENCES

These sources are provided for informational and educational purposes only. They support the scientific and physiological discussions presented in this book. Readers should always consult a qualified healthcare professional for personalized medical advice before implementing any peptide or wellness protocol.

Anderson, L. L., Smith, J. P., & Zhao, R. (2022). Peptide therapeutics: Progress and challenges. Nature Reviews Drug Discovery, 21(6), 421–439. https://doi.org/10.1038/s41573-022-00456-y

American College of Sports Medicine. (2021). ACSM's guidelines for exercise testing and prescription (11th ed.). Wolters Kluwer.

Bhasin, S., Brito, J. P., Cunningham, G. R., Hayes, F. J., & Wu, F. C. W. (2018). Testosterone therapy and muscle function in men: Clinical perspectives. Journal of Clinical Endocrinology & Metabolism, 103(11), 3963–3978. https://doi.org/10.1210/jc.2018-01374

Bjelakovic, G., Nikolova, D., Gluud, L. L., Simonetti, R. G., & Gluud, C. (2017). Antioxidant supplements for prevention of mortality in healthy participants and patients with various diseases. Cochrane Database of Systematic Reviews, 3, CD007176. https://doi.org/10.1002/14651858.CD007176.pub3

Boersma, G. J., Kalsbeek, A., & Fliers, E. (2020). Circadian rhythms and metabolic homeostasis. Current Opinion in Physiology, 15, 90–95. https://doi.org/10.1016/j.cophys.2020.03.003

Cadegiani, F. A., & Kater, C. E. (2020). Growth hormone secretagogues and body composition: A review. Frontiers in Endocrinology, 11, 419. https://doi.org/10.3389/fendo.2020.00419

Campbell, B. I., & Kreider, R. B. (2019). Protein intake and muscle maintenance during aging. Nutrients, 11(8), 1803. https://doi.org/10.3390/nu11081803

Centers for Disease Control and Prevention. (2023). Physical activity guidelines for adults. U.S. Department of Health and Human Services.

Datta, S. R., Horvath, T. L., & Sinclair, D. A. (2021). Mitochondrial peptides and longevity regulation. Cell Metabolism, 33(6), 1101–1113. https://doi.org/10.1016/j.cmet.2021.04.002

DiMarchi, R. D., & Enzmann, F. (2020). Peptide drug discovery and development. Annual Review of Pharmacology and Toxicology, 60, 25–44. https://doi.org/10.1146/annurev-pharmtox-010919-023604

Elahi, D., Nagamani, M., & Stewart, M. H. (2018). The role of ghrelin and growth hormone secretagogues in aging and metabolism. Endocrine Reviews, 39(3), 276–301. https://doi.org/10.1210/er.2017-00222

European Medicines Agency. (2022). Guidelines on peptide-based medicinal products. EMA.

Finan, B., Müller, T. D., Clemmensen, C., DiMarchi, R., & Tschöp, M. H. (2019). Unimolecular polyagonists for treatment of diabetes and obesity. Nature Medicine, 25(12), 173–180. https://doi.org/10.1038/s41591-019-0726-8

Forbes, S. C., & Bell, G. J. (2021). Resistance training and mitochondrial health. Sports Medicine, 51(4), 669–685. https://doi.org/10.1007/s40279-020-01393-5

Giordano, P., Rossi, F., & Gallo, C. (2019). Thymosin alpha 1: Immunomodulatory properties and clinical applications. Expert Opinion on Biological Therapy, 19(9), 923–932. https://doi.org/10.1080/14712598.2019.1636061

Goldman, A. M., & Berman, D. (2020). Integrative peptide therapies in regenerative medicine. Journal of Restorative Medicine, 9(1), 1–12. https://doi.org/10.14200/jrm.2020.0104

Gomez, D., Martinez, C., & Patel, K. (2023). KPV and intestinal inflammation: A novel therapeutic pathway. Peptides, 169, 170925. https://doi.org/10.1016/j.peptides.2023.170925

Hausenblas, H. A., & Cook, B. J. (2021). Exercise and mood enhancement: The role of neurochemistry. Frontiers in Psychology, 12, 615. https://doi.org/10.3389/fpsyg.2021.00615

He, F., Ouyang, D., & Yuan, L. (2020). Gut microbiota and metabolism in obesity and aging. Nutrients, 12(2), 345–357. https://doi.org/10.3390/nu12020345

Holzer, P., & Farzi, A. (2018). Neuropeptides and the microbiota–gut–brain axis. In Advances in Experimental Medicine and Biology (Vol. 1070, pp. 195–219). Springer.

International Peptide Society. (2023). Clinical applications of peptide therapeutics in metabolic and regenerative health [White paper].

Kalra, S. P. (2020). Neuroendocrine peptide control of appetite and energy balance. Physiology & Behavior, 227, 113143. https://doi.org/10.1016/j.physbeh.2020.113143

Laviano, A., Rossi Fanelli, F., & Muscaritoli, M. (2021). Protein, muscle, and aging: Nutritional interventions for longevity. Aging Clinical and Experimental Research, 33(9), 2387–2397. https://doi.org/10.1007/s40520-021-01881-8

Melmed, S., Kleinberg, D., & Ho, K. K. Y. (2019). Pituitary peptides and growth hormone signaling in health and disease. Endocrine Reviews, 40(3), 1109–1160. https://doi.org/10.1210/er.2018-00152

Miller, K. K., Zhou, J., & Sanders, J. (2020). Sleep peptides and circadian repair. Journal of Neuroendocrinology, 32(7), e12873. https://doi.org/10.1111/jne.12873

Myers, M. G., Jr. (2020). Selank and Semax: Peptide-based neuroprotective agents. Neuroscience Letters, 731, 135020. https://doi.org/10.1016/j.neulet.2020.135020

National Institutes of Health. (2022). Dietary protein and physical function in older adults. NIH Office of Nutrition Research.

Park, S. H., Lee, J. Y., & Choi, W. H. (2022). Epitalon and telomere preservation in aging models. Aging, 14(6), 2375–2390. https://doi.org/10.18632/aging.203990

Pavlov, V. A. (2020). Neuropeptides, inflammation, and the gut-brain axis. Peptides, 132, 170348. https://doi.org/10.1016/j.peptides.2020.170348

Pottel, L., Rombouts, S., & De Bruyn, M. (2021). GHK-Cu peptide in wound healing and skin regeneration. Journal of Cosmetic Dermatology, 20(8), 2609–2617. https://doi.org/10.1111/jocd.13968

Riera, C. E., & Dillin, A. (2019). Peptide hormones and aging control. Nature Reviews Molecular Cell Biology, 20(5), 275–290. https://doi.org/10.1038/s41580-018-0087-8

Sakellariou, G. K., Pearson, T., & Jackson, M. J. (2019). Muscle recovery and mitochondrial peptides. Experimental Gerontology, 118, 132–142. https://doi.org/10.1016/j.exger.2019.01.019

Sinha, R., Davis, S. N., & Polonsky, K. S. (2023). GLP-1 receptor agonists: Metabolic modulation and weight control. New England Journal of Medicine, 388(10), 910–921. https://doi.org/10.1056/NEJMra2209843

Smith, J. P., Smithson, A., & Pavlov, V. A. (2021). BPC-157: Mechanisms of tissue repair and clinical applications. Current Pharmaceutical Design, 27(36), 3764–3775. https://doi.org/10.2174/1381612827666210429114240

Spierings, E. L. H., de Vries, M., & Leenders, F. (2020). Thymosin beta 4 and angiogenesis in tissue regeneration. Peptide Science, 112(5), e24190. https://doi.org/10.1002/pep2.24190

Thorner, M. O., Ho, K. K. Y., & Melmed, S. (2018). Clinical use of growth hormone–releasing hormone analogs. Endocrine Practice, 24(9), 839–848. https://doi.org/10.4158/EP-2018-0192

Toth, A. E., Nielsen, K., & Petersen, M. A. (2022). Peptide-based therapies for neurological disorders. Frontiers in Pharmacology, 13, 845217. https://doi.org/10.3389/fphar.2022.845217

United States Food and Drug Administration. (2024). Guidelines for compounding and handling peptide biologics. U.S. Department of Health and Human Services.

Volpe, S. L. (2021). Hydration, electrolytes, and performance in midlife adults. ACSM's Health & Fitness Journal, 25(5), 22–30. https://doi.org/10.1249/FIT.0000000000000669

World Health Organization. (2023). Healthy aging and physical activity: Global recommendations. WHO.

Made in the USA
Monee, IL
11 November 2026

cb0764e8-65a5-4a83-b700-590ef0ea20a8R01